D0276640

EVERYTHING THAT MAKES US HUMAN

EVERYTHING THAT MAKES US HUMAN

Case Notes of a Children's Brain Surgeon

JAY JAYAMOHAN

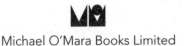

Michael O'Mara Books Limited

For my family

First published in Great Britain in 2020 by
Michael O'Mara Books Limited
9 Lion Yard
Tremadoc Road
London SW4 7NQ

Copyright © Jayaratnam Jayamohan 2020
Text written by Jeff Hudson 2020
Text copyright © Michael O'Mara Books Ltd 2020

All rights reserved. You may not copy, store, distribute, transmit, reproduce or otherwise make available this publication (or any part of it) in any form, or by any means (electronic, digital, optical, mechanical, photocopying, recording or otherwise), without the prior written permission of the publisher. Any person who does any unauthorized act in relation to this publication may be liable to criminal prosecution and civil claims for damages.

A CIP catalogue record for this book is available from the British Library.

Papers used by Michael O'Mara Books Limited are natural, recyclable products made from wood grown in sustainable forests. The manufacturing processes conform to the environmental regulations of the country of origin.

Some names and identifying details have been changed to protect the privacy of individuals.

ISBN: 978-1-78929-140-7 in hardback print format
ISBN: 978-1-78929-154-4 in ebook format

2 3 4 5 6 7 8 9 10

Designed and typeset by Claire Cater
Printed and bound by CPI Group (UK) Ltd, Croydon, CR0 4YY
www.mombooks.com

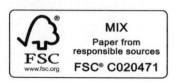

MIX
Paper from
responsible sources
FSC
www.fsc.org
FSC® C020471

CONTENTS

DO NO HARM

Uh. Uh-uh-uh. Uh-uh-uh. Uh. Uh. Uh. Uh.

The opening chords of AC/DC's 'Back in Black' ring out. The image of Angus Young – the band's guitarist in trademark schoolboy uniform – flick fleetingly across my mind. Very fleetingly.

The large screens behind me are in focus, ready to go. I look at the anaesthetist. She gives me the nod. I check with the scrub nurse. She's primed, prepped. Ready.

Finally, I look down at the tiny bundle of humanity on the table beneath me. I pick up my knife and I say, 'Let's begin.'

· · ◆ · ·

Ever since I was little, music has meant a lot. When I was nine, my uncle gave me a cheap Pye tape recorder. I used it to do what I imagine everybody my age did back then, which was to tape the Top 40 singles chart. I realized that when I was listening to that, the rest of the world faded away and I was able to concentrate. Everything just stuck when the volume was up. I could do my homework and read books so much more easily. Through O levels, A levels and medical school, if I didn't have my headphones on then nothing was sinking in. There was too much extraneous noise. I was too easily distracted.

And in an operating theatre with an eighteen-month-old baby in front of you, distracted is the last thing you can afford to be. For their sake and yours, you want and need to be at the top of your game. It's the only way to stack the odds against whatever is attacking them. Tumour, spina bifida, massive head trauma. I – we – can try to fight them all. But only when I'm concentrating.

I don't always win. I can't always win. But I try. I do everything possible to abide by the number-one rule in the doctors' handbook, and the title of a book written by one of my old teachers and inspirations, Henry Marsh: do no harm. And then some. And that's what I tell the patients and their parents when they come to the question they always eventually ask: 'Doctor Jay, tell us. What are the odds?'

They can't help it. They want to know, in terms they can understand, just how likely it is that their child will survive. How certain that the operation their loved one is about to undergo will be successful. They want a percentage, a number out of 100. Something they can translate. Something they can process.

I'm no mathematician, but I do my best. I'm always honest. I always reply. Sometimes the win/lose ratio is 50:50. Sometimes it's 90:10. Sometimes it's the opposite way round.

It doesn't really matter. I always follow up with the same words: 'I can tell you the odds, but whether there's a five per cent or a ninety-five per cent chance of success, it doesn't matter. We're going to go for it. We're going to do our best.'

The 'we' means all of us – doctors, nurses, scrub staff and, of course, parents and patients. Because the alternative doesn't bear thinking about.

I became a doctor to save lives. I became a neurosurgeon because I believed it to be the highest achievement in medicine. I became a paediatric neurosurgeon to give a voice to those patients so long overlooked because of their age. To give them a life. To give them a chance. To give them respect.

· · ◆ · ·

In the background my young registrar flicks the volume dial on the speaker.

UH. UH-UH-UH. UH-UH-UH. UH. UH. UH. UH.

'Let's do this.'

CHAPTER ONE

HOLY MOLY

It's 7.45 a.m. Surgery day. Time to meet the contestants.

The pre-operative ward is – I like to think in my egotistical way – a bit like the airlock chamber in a spacecraft. It prepares you for what's to come. I'm there with a junior trainee neurosurgeon plus a couple of young doctors, the core of the team soon to go to work. To be honest, it's more of a courtesy call than anything, as the patient and her family have seen us all before. We've already gone through the procedure at length during clinic and then again over the last few days. In the week before an operation, I like patients to come in beforehand to be assessed by the whole team of specialists. Nobody stays over unless they're too ill to move. They get checked and double-checked by everyone who I think can offer some insight. I prefer to keep surprises during the operating process down to a minimum.

These eleventh-hour visits are mainly to check that the little one hasn't developed a chest infection or anything overnight and to make sure there are no last-minute questions from anyone. It's also the last chance that parents and patient get to meet the team before we dive behind our face masks. It's important to me that they know exactly who is looking after their pride and joy.

Finally, we get a few confirmation signatures – 'You accept the risks, any more questions?' – and we're ready. All the big conversations have been had on previous days. I ensure that they hear the standard Jayamohan promise: I will treat their child as I would want my own kids treated if they were sick. No bigger promise exists, in my opinion.

If we have our timing right we should run into the rest of the team for ward rounds at exactly 8 o'clock. We have four neurosurgeons, two or three plastic surgery consultants who work alongside us, a smattering of juniors – a couple of registrars and ward doctors – a nurse or two, plus the odd medical student. It can turn into a large crowd.

I'm sure it can be quite intimidating to have a John Radcliffe XI surround your bed, especially if you're barely old enough to fill a third of it, but I hope it conveys the right message: we're here to help. All of us.

Babies tend to treat it as they do everything else, with sleepy indifference. They're like cats but less fickle. Parents, on the other hand, don't know where to look, let alone stand.

No patient is more important than another – except on surgery days. At 8.30 a.m. I break off from the general meet 'n' greets and make my way to theatre.

You see sportsmen and women often get into a huddle before a big match. For them it's a sign of public solidarity. The Team vs The World. When we do it, it's more about making sure that we don't chop out the wrong bit of the brain.

Before every operation these days we tick off the 'WHO' – the surgery checklist introduced by the World Health Organization to eradicate errors. It's so simple, yet so effective.

Patients are already booked in on our electronic system, to let the scrub nurses know what we'll be doing and which kit needs to be prepared. Everyone about to be involved in the forthcoming operation introduces themselves to the others. Nine times out of ten we know each other anyway, but new trainees or nurses do appear every so often. Research shows that even knowing everyone's name and role can reduce errors.

Next, we'll talk about the patients. Whoever the 'lead' is will give a quick, short version of the history and map out what we're planning to do. If I'm there it usually means I'm the lead. On cases that are predominantly cranial or facial reconstruction, then a colleague from plastic surgery will step forward. We talk about what equipment we need. We check with the nurses that they have all the tools that we have requested previously. We go around the room and just get that verbal guarantee that there are no issues or concerns.

If I have any pointers, I'll call them out. For example, 'the main issue today is going to be blood loss' or 'the key concern for this case will be post-operative infection, so let's make sure the doors are shut, there are no students in the room and no one walks in and out'. It's all common sense, but it bears repeating.

One of the premises of WHO is to make everyone feel equal so that the most junior member of staff is able to question what the most senior person is doing. From my point of view, being the most senior surgeon in most operating rooms, that could get quite annoying quite quickly, but the logic is sound. If we've said we're going to do an operation on the left side of the head and if a student watches us about to start an operation on the right, then they need to feel comfortable enough to say, 'Excuse me, Doctor Jay, but I'm pretty sure you said the left side of the head.'

Trust me, it's happened elsewhere – otherwise they wouldn't introduce a rule about it.

If everyone is satisfied about what's to follow, we break off. While most of us go back to finish off our ward rounds, the anaesthetist then calls for the patient. What happens next depends on how long it takes for the patient to be prepared for the anaesthetic and then be put 'under'. The longer the anaesthetist takes to prep, the happier I am. In forty minutes I can squeeze in about ten patient visits. It's all about spinning as many plates as possible at once.

If I'm the guy leading the operation – and today I am – I'll peel away from the ward before the others finish. If it's one of my neuro patients, I like to get ready and be in the room before they're completely under.

Each set of operating theatres has its own changing area. I strip down to my underwear and pull on my blues and surgical shoes. For reasons of hygiene, the blues get boil-washed by the hospital, so they smell like everything else in the building. They are available in four different sizes, which in theory is enough to fit every shape. In practice, however, 'no size fits anyone' would be more accurate.

The shoes look like uglier versions of Crocs, but if you get the right pair they're super comfortable. I tend to squirrel away my ones in my locker. If I left them out, someone would pinch them – probably a student. When you're on your feet for seven or eight hours it's important not to be hopping from foot to foot. We used to have a dishwasher that was bastardized into a shoe washer, but we don't anymore. You have to clean your own shoes now.

Medicine isn't the ideal game for anyone with sensitive skin. By 9.30 a.m., I've probably washed my hands fifteen to twenty times. Every time you touch a patient, you wash; before you touch a patient, you wash; in between, you wash out of habit. You're just constantly scrubbing or disinfecting.

It's nearly show time. The quickest way into the operating theatre is via the anaesthetist's room. Generally, out of respect for his or her workspace, we'll use the doors at the back. The patient will be wheeled through from next door when the time is right.

The theatre is probably about 5 metres by 5 metres or thereabouts. It's all designed around the space for the table in the middle. You could plonk me in any hospital and I probably couldn't tell them apart. They're all lined with the same boring melamine-type walls that can easily be sterilized and washed down. They have a set of lights in the roof and the various pipes and cables that send around oxygen and other gases, and suck away all the unwanted leftovers of an operation – blood, mucous, saliva, and other slip hazards. Most of the equipment is portable. It gets wheeled in and out as and when required.

Today, we have the anaesthetic machine at the foot of the bed – obviously, since I'm working on the other end. Then we've got a few bits of kit, like suction and electrocautery (a means of using electricity to literally cut tissue – the closest to a real-life light sabre that exists, I think), sitting on a large trolley at the end of the table as well. Four computers are scattered around for maximum access. We'll put the scans up on the large screens, conduct electronic monitoring of the patient and provide notes for the anaesthetist. That is if all the machines are working …

You only have to have one failure at a crucial time for you never to trust any piece of technology again. And it's just as well we checked.

'Jay, I can only see one of these screens working,' says my assistant. I'm no Bill Gates, but I take a look anyway. 'Do you think it's the machine or the screen?'

'Not a clue.'

'Do me a favour – go and swap it with Theatre Twelve.'

'Oh, come on. I did it last time.'

'You bloody didn't – *I* was the one nearly caught, not you.'

Oh, the joys of the NHS … I'm not sure why our machine doesn't work. I suspect that one of the other theatres switched their duff one with ours, so it's only fair if we steal a working one back. I do usually try to send one of the juniors, but I'm not above a little light-fingered jiggery-pokery myself.

With all the machines that go 'ping' in place, we load up the scans and once again I'll talk the team through our aims and hopes. Depending on when you meet them, registrars can be box fresh or have up to eight years' surgical experience, so it's good to know who's who. Of course, I know the more senior ones, but usually you can work it out. The novices ask dozens of questions and the older ones just want to grab your tools and do everything themselves. It's not unknown for them to try to steal patients from me. As a speciality there's probably more work performed by consultants in paediatric neurosurgery than in other disciplines, for the simple reason that things can go pear-shaped so much more quickly. But I do try to encourage and involve where I can. As soon as the scans are loaded, I ask the registrar's opinion of what we're about to embark upon.

The final check is with the nurses, or 'scrubs' as surgical specialists are called. You'll have seen the big tray of shiny silver implements on TV. Based on what they know of my plans, everything on the tray should be ready and waiting.

'Does this look okay, Jay?' the lead scrub asks. It would be unprofessional of me not to check, but I know everything I could possibly need will be there. I look down at the 250 or so instruments. It's quite the expensive toolbox. We have different-sized clips, different-sized scalpel holders, different-sized 'rakes' and retractors – tools used to pull tissue out of the way with; some sharp, some blunt. We have bone nibblers – instruments like pliers that will bite off or 'nibble' bone; brain retractors – lollipop sticks that range in size from ginormous to tiny, which you can use to move the brain out of the way; spatulas; suckers; scissors, from the very big for cutting heavy tissue or stitches, through to micro-scissors, which are tiny. We have tools for probing, for pushing, for pulling, for poking, for cutting, for grabbing. It's pretty impressive.

Once all the checks are done, we're ready to go. All we need now is our star attraction. If it's a quick anaesthetic on a small case that doesn't need lots of drips, catheters and other pipes inserted, it may be fifteen or twenty minutes before the patient is signed off as ready. If it's a bigger sort of operation, like a tumour removal, or if the patient has an abnormal anatomy, it could take as long as ninety minutes to get prepped. The anaesthetist isn't just responsible for pain and consciousness management; he or she will have blood ready in case of significant loss. Their job is essentially to keep the patient alive while I work at the other end.

Eventually, the doors swing open and the patient arrives. I have a quick chat with the anaesthetist again to make sure everything is still okay. Then we scoop the patient from the anaesthetic trolley onto the operating table itself, and spend serious time getting them positioned properly. Operations can take seven or eight hours. Patients need to be able to lie still for that long without long-lasting effects. If they're lying on a wire or a hard catheter, after eight hours that can actually kill the skin. We pack their body with lots of swabs and gauzes, and nowadays we also use a special memory foam which cuddles the patient and gives them a really nice, soft, yielding surface to lie on.

We also need to ensure that we have easy access. We know exactly where we want to operate, but we have to be able to get into that area safely and easily, and think about whether we want to stand or sit during the operation. All of these permutations go through my head prior to commencing the surgery.

The one thing I don't have to worry about is the team around me. There's an element of 'emergency' about neurosurgery; plenty of what we do happens in response to a 999 call. When it does, it's all hands on deck. At least it should be. I've worked with anaesthetists and trainees who, to be frank, loved the job and were very good at it between the hours of nine to five. But I've had to steel myself plenty of times to phone certain people in the middle of the night, knowing they'll not be that interested. When it's 3 o'clock in the morning and you're dead on your feet, what really doesn't help is if somebody's got a face like a wet weekend. It's not a great vibe for life-or-death work. I'd rather have the guys who bite my head off and get it out of their system, then crack on as normal. Or, ideally, the ones who recognize that this is a team effort, that we are there to help the patient. That we aren't operating in the middle of the night because there's nothing on the telly.

All the while we've been prepping, the sounds of my Spotify techno-dance playlist are echoing around the room. I've got a different playlist for different procedures. Downstairs, where we tend to work more on facial reconstruction, we play more rock music, but that's because the plastics guys can't cope with too much electronica. Upstairs, where we are now, and about to tackle a tumour with a difference, techno and dance seem to help me to work better. Something about the beats per minute lets me zone out of the real world, so I'm only seeing the work. But you never know until you get going.

And finally, we're ready.

Our patient is a one-year-old girl with a brain tumour that's taking up half of her head. It's unusual to say the least. Not because tumours can't grow to hideous proportions – but because she doesn't seem to have noticed. It really is incredible. I've seen the CT scans and the MRIs plenty of times. Even so, looking at them projecting from the computer, I'm shaking my head as I did the first time I saw it.

She first came to our attention at eight weeks old. The obvious action back then was to schedule tumour surgery. Get the bugger out. But despite being malignant, the tumour seemed to be largely inactive. By a stroke of luck, it was growing out of the brain and compressing it – rather than invading deep inside. To look at the scans you wouldn't see a jumbled mess of interwoven strands; more like the half-and-half design of the yin and yang symbols. Two things growing side by side, like two people in the back of a small car – uncomfortable, but not interfering.

Years ago, when I started out, I would not have bet a penny on her still being alive today. But that's because I'd rarely seen a tumour play so nicely before. To be fair, the brain should take its share of the credit. Because the tumour started throwing its weight around *in utero*, before she was even born, the girl's brain has been

17

adapting ever since. You normally put control of the left-hand side of the body over there? Tough. That space is taken. How about we squeeze it in here? It has literally relocated important nerve centres to more convenient places. The ability for children's brains to rewire and reorganize themselves is remarkable. They have this amazing aptitude for plasticity. Trust me: any adult would have died a long, long time ago. Our brains get too fixed in their ways. This girl is a living, evolving masterpiece.

Even so, enough is enough. At the current rate of growth, our patient will soon find her brain compressed dramatically. Serious cerebral dysfunction will surely follow.

It's one of the cleanest ops I've ever done. Four hours later and we have managed to remove the tumour virtually in its entirety. What's left is a cavern, a space where usually half a fully grown brain would be. And yet not one important controlling function has been impacted. It looks weird, crazy even, but with all the nerve tissue still intact in the small half that's left, it's going to be business as usual almost as soon as she wakes up. And it was, almost. Just a tiny bit of weakness in one side, which got better and didn't seem to affect her life.

Six years later, every time I see that little girl, it's such a great feeling to think, *Holy moly, I thought you were going to be dead within six months.* Not only is she not dead, but she's awesome. And she'll certainly outlive me. Not that she knows who I am. To her I'm just the annoying man who bangs a small hammer on her knee once a year and bombards her with questions. I'm probably a right pain in her backside.

But do you know what? That's fine with me. I'd take that result every single time.

CHAPTER TWO

CALL ME 'MISTER'

The hands. It always starts with the hands.

It's funny, really. A child might be at death's door. As far as the parents are aware, I am the person who stands a chance of bringing their bundle of joy back from the brink. I've been doing this my entire adult life. I've saved hundreds of children with the exact same symptoms. But sometimes it doesn't cross their minds to check that. They don't ask for my CV. They don't enquire about past success rates. They stare at my hands.

Does he have the hands of someone who could save our child?

I get it. I'm going to be putting my fingers inside their baby's skull. Touching its brain, most likely. They want assurances that I'm worthy, that I'm not shaking, that I'm *clean*. We scrub our hands thoroughly before we operate, and of course we wear gloves for all procedures. There was a short-lived attempt to suggest that we only needed to do a full 'surgical scrub' – the kind you see on the telly – in the morning, and then just a simple handwash between each case that day. It didn't happen, despite the evidence that was presented to us. Some things can't be changed – surgeons and nurses have their routines, and we need to do them to keep our anxiety at bay.

But it's all about appearances. And appearances where desperate parents are concerned count for more than you think. It's a lesson I've learned over more than fifteen years as a consultant and almost double that time as a doctor.

And yet not everyone sets great store on such things. Not everyone even notices what parents think. Some people, in fact, couldn't care less. Which is why I am the man I am today and why I choose to work with children. And which is why I try to go the extra mile and place myself in not just the parents' shoes, but those of my patients. How would I feel in their position? What would make my already horrific ordeal that bit better?

I like to think that I do what I can, and should, for my patients. But it wasn't always like that. And it certainly wasn't what I was always taught.

At the age of eighteen I went off to medical school. I chose St Mary's in Paddington, London. I had thought about Oxford – my biology teacher said that this was clearly where I should go – but after having visited it, I felt that it seemed too quiet, too provincial for the teenage me. I wanted the grubby highlights of the big smoke. Interesting how this view was to change later on in my life. Six years of medical school is a long time, but you soon realize after qualification that even half a century of study would have left you feeling you had gaps in your knowledge. All these years later I'm still learning. Of course, that's with the benefit of hindsight. At that age you think you know it all.

I was bright-eyed and bushy tailed, full of enthusiasm and enough confidence to think I could change the world. A typical eighteen-year-old, in other words. It was a bit of a shock to learn that the whole profession had slightly lower aspirations. The father of modern medicine, Hippocrates himself, summed it up in a nutshell: 'Do no harm.' (Well, he didn't actually make it up, but let's not quibble – it simply paraphrased his 'oath' that doctors love so much.) In other words, don't screw up. That's it. That's all doctors were expected to do. Don't make things worse. Anything better than that is a bonus. Surely, we must have moved on from there?

Reality check aside, the course covered everything, and as much as it makes me sound nerdy, I liked it all. Whichever topic we covered that week became my new life's ambition. I was like a kitten chasing beams of light. *Ooh, sparkly. Ooh, new! Want it, chase it, want it.*

It was only as we went through year five that I decided upon my future speciality. Or so I thought. In your penultimate year of being a medical student, essentially after nearly six years of hard slog and excessive drinking, they throw you a bone. You're asked to do a three-month specialism with the bonus of the powers-that-be letting you choose where to do it. Most people pick Jamaica or Thailand or Australia, basically somewhere to chill.

I chose the National Hospital for Neurology and Neurosurgery in Queen Square in London. Just down the road. What a loser.

In my defence, they had a great reputation for my new favourite topic: neurology, the medical side of brain disorders. The passion had been growing for some time. Lots of people have a model of that phrenology bust on their shelves – the human head with the various parts of the brain marked off like prime cuts on a picture of a cow. You'd be forgiven for thinking that it is an accurate representation of what's under the hood – and certainly in the early 19th century most experts did – but it's largely inaccurate. Having said that, as incredible as it sounds, there are some areas of the brain that were successfully associated with specific functions as far back as ancient Egyptian times.

An American collector of antiquities called Edwin Smith discovered an almost 4,000-year-old papyrus containing a fantastic collection of descriptions of what are clearly neurosurgical wounds alongside explanations of what should be done to make them better. Things like: 'If the man has a wound to his temple, and cannot speak, this is a wound that cannot be treated', because they obviously knew that the speech centres were in these areas. It lists different presentations of spinal injuries and gives a spookily accurate assessment of the prognosis for each. There are lots of nuggets like these, all born thousands of years ago from, one imagines, observations of people with battle injuries. It's fascinating to consider the physicians working independently, but all their information has been pulled together over time. One doctor would look at a patient and say, 'Okay, you can't move. There's a hole in this part of your head, so they must be connected.' He would write that down and over time people would build on that knowledge.

Like so many advancements in science and technology today, the driving factor has been the effects of war rather than a thirst for health. But the ancient Egyptians weren't the only ones on record to dabble in neurosurgery. There's evidence from over 3,000 years ago in Central and South America, where they used to trepan – in other words, drill holes in skulls to let out the evil humours. It's almost inconceivable that there was neurosurgery going on back then, but the fact that there was further sold it to me as a worthwhile career.

The great thing about any neurological condition, though, and this is why I was drawn to it, is that it takes a lot of thought. It's a very deductive speciality. You examine patients, and you have to work out where the problem lies, at what level and which part of the function of that person is affected. It's like doing a cryptic crossword. The clues are there, but can you make sense of them? You're Dr Watson and Sherlock Holmes rolled into one. I absolutely loved it. It spoke to me. Challenged me. And, I guess, didn't exactly hurt my ego.

It's not for everyone. Many of my friends were drawn to orthopaedics. I wasn't going to judge them, but where was the challenge in that? 'You've got a broken leg. Here's an X-ray, it shows me the leg is broken. Job done.'

Of course, now I know that orthopaedics can be incredibly intricate and challenging, but I didn't see that side of these specialities back then – you only get two to three months at most, and sometimes much less, at medical school.

I didn't want something that would give me answers on a plate. I wanted to have to sit and think and work stuff out. Be a calculator rather than a robot on the production line. But, I began to wonder, would that be enough?

The thing about Sherlock, of course, is that while he was the greatest deductive detective, he was also, like the Dark Knight, no slouch at the old fisticuffs. He could handle the practical as well as the theoretical side of crime-solving. Whereas I, in neurology, was being benched whenever the going got good. The problem with neurology as a discipline is that although it's really good for all that deductive reasoning, the treatment options can be limited. I felt slightly powerless in that I was going to be giving patients some medicine and seeing if the medicine helped, rather than me helping personally. I may as well have been standing on that weird raised step in a pharmacy doling out ibuprofen for all the input I thought I'd be giving. It didn't feel like I was actually part of the treatment – just a conduit for the drugs. I think it was all part of a rather youthful desire to be the centre of everything.

But, I reasoned, *so what if I rarely break a sweat? This is the area I want to specialize in.*

By the third month, however, it had got to me. I was in the dining hall at Queen Square queuing for something with chips, whatever the day's special was, and I remember ranting to a couple of friends about the shortcomings of the area.

'I never feel like I *do* anything. I got into medicine to help people, not read books. I want to get my hands dirty.' I was talking to a group of neurology hopefuls, so I wasn't going to get any sympathy from them. Nor, it turned out, from anyone else.

'Stop fucking whingeing,' said a voice from behind me. I turned to see that, according to his name tag, it was one of the university's senior trainee neurosurgeons. 'If you really want to get your hands dirty then stop moaning and do something about it. Join us. Be a brain surgeon. Ditch these losers. Become one of the elite.'

I don't think I moved for about a minute as I was so shocked at being sworn at like that by a stranger. By the time I did, the lunch queue had shifted around me and the guy was already at the till. I was torn between grabbing the chilli option and running after him. In the end I tried to do both. Clutching my food, I chucked a fiver at the cashier and legged it after my new mentor. So what if he eavesdropped on other people's conversations? I liked the cut of the guy's jib. He had this arrogance I'd never seen in doctors before. It was intoxicating. It spoke to me. He was exactly everything I wanted to be.

'Do yourself a favour,' he said, barely looking at me when I caught up. 'Come and see what we do. You've either got it or you haven't.' He explained that he was operating the following day and I was welcome to attend.

Eighteen hours later, I was watching him cut into a young woman's head. I needed to become one of these guys. Of course I did. It was so obvious. This guy wasn't just deducing the problem and prescribing a few pills. He was nailing the diagnostic bit and then providing the solution with his own two hands.

He's not just dishing out the medicine. He *is* the medicine.

My future was fixed at that very moment. But before I got there, despite what it said at my graduation ceremony about being qualified, I needed to learn to become a *real* doctor.

All the theory in the world can't prepare you for what lies outside the college doors. After qualifying, you used to do a year's basic medicine and surgery, basically a bit of everything, before you could even think of sub-specializing. In other words, you're let loose on the public. Again I eschewed the glamour spots of the world for Ealing Hospital. Like all newbies, I thought I had all the answers.

Like all newbies, I was soon put in my place. I knew nothing.

There was six months of general surgery and another six of general medicine. That's really when you learn how to be a doctor. And it's a steep learning curve. During my first 'on-call' shift as a doctor, I was asked to 'write up' some paracetamol. There happened to be a box near me in the drug cupboard, so I broke a couple of tablets out and handed them over.

'What are you doing, lad?' the nurse in charge asked. 'You can't just hand out medicine. You have to prescribe it.'

'Okay,' I said, and I duly wrote down 'two paracetamol'. 'There you go.'

She rolled her eyes and laughed. 'You can't write "two tablets". You have to write "one gram".'

'Really? Six years and no one told me that?'

'That's why you're here.'

Measuring tablets in weight was just the start of it. There were so many idiosyncrasies not covered in the textbooks and of course the only way to learn was to have first-hand experience. I examined hundreds of patients, processed thousands of blood tests, listened to countless heartbeats. It was baffling how so many people of the same species suffering the same conditions could have such different bodies. At med school all the practice dummies looked the same. Still, all part of the learning process.

The lack of time and resources in the NHS means there's no room for slowcoaches. As nice as most people were, carrying a newbie passenger wasn't something anyone enjoyed. They made that clear enough. And why not? They'd had to get up to speed sharpish back in the day. There was no reason I shouldn't either.

You had to learn quickly. There just wasn't the time for anything else. I was basically only shown anything once. If it didn't stick, you didn't dare ask again. The whole culture was summarized succinctly by one of the doctors in the following words: 'See one, do one, teach one.' That was workable when you were writing out prescriptions.

When we moved onto the surgery half of the year, the risks got a little higher and Hippocrates' words finally made sense. You're dealing with someone's internal organs. It's not Lego, it's not Stickle Bricks. If anything it's Jenga. One slip and you can wreck everything. Surgeons aren't magicians. As one of them said, 'We don't deal in miracles. If in doubt, do nothing at all.'

Do no harm.

Every fledgling doctor has to pass the whole year. Whether you're aspiring to become a GP, a gynaecologist or the future of oncology, it all begins with this cold immersion into reality. These days it's spread out over two years. Even double that, I would suggest, couldn't begin to prepare you comfortably for the world outside.

The surgery aspect only confirmed my decision to focus on neurosurgery, but I still had two more years of hurdles to overcome before I could even begin. Now promoted to Senior House Officer, 'Dr Jay' was expected to turn his hand to everything at the hospital of his choice and I elected Kingston in Surrey.

My first stint was in A&E. If I thought doling out painkillers was an ordeal, then this was something else. If you've ever gone into A&E and thought the treating doctor looked a little scared, you're right. I honestly didn't know what I was doing quite a lot of the time. If you gave me rare and seemingly random symptoms as part of an exam, I'd ace it. 'Erratic behaviour in a patient with sweet smelling urine and ear wax? That must be a metabolic condition known as branched-chain ketoaciduria. I think that patient is suffering from Maple syrup urine disease, sir.' (That's a real thing, by the way.)

But staring into the eyes of a real-life human being at 1 o'clock on a Sunday morning, trying to unpack the truth from the confused guesses the patient has made about his or her condition, the pressure was slightly different. So many variables, so many red herrings. Thankfully, there are the nurses. These people saved my backside countless times, and are the absolute backbone of the department. An experienced A&E nurse is worth more than sleep – and that was something I was sorely lacking.

A&E really is the front line of medicine. You're firefighting all the time. It's a really worthy part of the system, but it wasn't where I wanted to be. Nor was general surgery nor orthopaedic surgery, even after six months doing each. *No*, I thought, *my future is in neurosurgery. I want to be a 'Mr'.*

It's a weird quirk of UK medicine – certainly it's viewed as weird by international colleagues and, if I'm honest, most of my patients – that once you qualify as a surgeon you are elevated beyond the soubriquet of 'doctor'. As a breed we're quite passionate about the origins of the tradition. Like so many British oddities it has its roots in snobbery.

To be a doctor in the 1700s required a medical degree. In theory, this was a sign of erudition. In practice, degrees were often acquired by charlatans cheaply, abroad or by post. It didn't matter, as it bestowed upon them the title of 'Dr' and the right to prescribe medicines, albeit from a rather narrow range, and charge bills. Big bills.

Occasionally, their diagnosis would require some bloodletting or bone-cutting, which is where the surgeon would come in. Except in those days, surgeons weren't considered medical men. Far from it. They were butchers or, more accurately, barbers.

If you needed a bladder stone removed or a tooth yanked out, you'd be sent along to the same place where you got your hair cut. This is why, if you look outside barbershops today, you'll often see a pole of red-and-white stripes. It signifies the blood and bandages of their forefathers' 'other' jobs.

It was considered such a ghastly side of health care that doctors weren't going to perform surgery themselves. All that blood and gore was considered beneath them. Not only were surgeons not required to have qualifications as doctors, all they really needed was muscle, something no man of learning would possess. If a doctor diagnosed a gangrenous foot, for example, then your local Vidal Sassoon would basically stick a leather strap in your mouth and four big blokes would hold you down while the barber got the saw out. Doctors wanted absolutely nothing to do with it.

It was only in the 1800s, with the advent of antisepsis and some element of anaesthetic, that surgery began to lose its tag of human torture and people would voluntarily go to the surgeon and say, 'I think there's something wrong with me.' As it evolved as an occupation and became more skilled and more licensed – and less deadly – the medical profession made moves to bring this former black sheep of the family under its own roof, which of course made sense. But even as they became 'legit' members of the industry, surgeons wanted nothing to do with those quacks who'd once treated them like dog mess on their shoes, so they refused the title of 'Dr'. And which is why, out of solidarity with our predecessors, surgeons in the UK still do the same today. Myself included.

After six years of struggle to become a 'Dr', I couldn't wait to get rid of it.

It was at a hospital in leafy Wimbledon where I finally got my chance to practise neurosurgery and, from the moment I passed my junior surgeon exams, my title changed as well. It gave me an inordinate amount of pleasure to ask people to 'Call me "Mister".' It sounds really childish, but this title had cost me so much time and effort, and all the surgeons I knew got a kick out of this name change.

I worked with half a dozen neurosurgeons, some more closely than others. They were a mix of consultants and senior trainees who were basically at the end of their training. They all had their strengths and weaknesses. Some would let me do more than run errands and watch them in theatre, but they might be unpleasant personally. Others were charm personified, but always, I felt, holding me back from contributing anything worthwhile. What they all had in common, however, was this unerring belief that they were operating – pun intended – at the top of the medical profession. The swagger wasn't just reserved for the guy at Queen Square who'd helped to change my career path. They all had it coursing through them. As one of them admitted to me during an operation, 'All doctors have a God complex – but we're the only ones who deserve it.'

I could see what they meant. Your heart is important but, at the end of the day, it's basically a pump. A fancy irrigation system. Whereas the brain is network control. You want anything done, speak to the brain – oh wait, you can't because the brain controls speech.

I admit it. I was falling for the hype hook, line and sinker. In the meantime, my big brother was training to be a heart surgeon. We had a vague sort of competition going on between our specialities. He never gave an inch. Never doubted his side of the great divide. And, when we both experienced one of his colleagues close up, I could see why.

· · ◆ · ·

I still remember the day I got the call from my dad telling me that he required a triple heart bypass. He was youngish, relatively fit and had never smoked, so it was a shock. Despite all three of us being in the medical game, the waiting list for Dad's operation was some months *after* they predicted he would likely suffer a heart attack. That seemed a bit back to front. Fortunately, Dad had health insurance. I'd never understood why a doctor would get insurance but, given the waiting-list issues, it was all suddenly clear – he knew exactly what pressures the NHS was under and, given the predictions, we all knew this was the only way to go. So, given that we were paying, my cardiac surgery trainee brother knew exactly who he wanted to conduct the operation.

On the morning of the operation, my brother and I were at the hospital to give moral support to my mum. Dad was in bullish spirits and, as he was wheeled away, so was I. As the hours passed, that confidence began to slip. Despite all my training, the thought of a stranger with his hands inside our dad's chest was unsettling.

I remember asking my brother, 'I know you were his registrar, but are you sure about this guy?'

'I've told you,' he said. 'He's the best. You wouldn't want anyone else.'

'Let's hope you're right.'

It was a long and painful five hours of waiting and waiting. I must have covered every inch of the floor in the first sixty minutes alone. Apart from a quick dash down to the supermarket in the lobby, the rest of the time I'd spent gazing absent-mindedly out of the window. Eventually, though, I had to ask, 'What's taking so long?'

'I'm sure everything is fine,' my brother said. 'They're just being thorough.'

'Yeah, I suppose you're right. You wouldn't want them to rush – hey! Wait a minute.' I called him over to the window. 'Is that who I think it is?'

A few floors down below was the unmistakable figure of my father's surgeon, climbing into a car. 'What the hell's he doing out there?' I asked.

'He must have finished,' he replied.

'And he didn't bother to come and tell us how it went? You were his fucking registrar!'

Despite his defence of the guy, my brother was just as offended as I was that no contact had been made. We'd been waiting for nearly six hours and literally didn't know where our dad was, alive or not. I'd had enough. I went running down the hall and was just about to give someone a piece of my mind when the anaesthetist from the operation walked out. He too had been handpicked.

'There you are,' he said. 'I was just coming to find you.'

'Is Dad all right?' I asked.

'Should be fine. The next twenty-four hours, as you know, are crucial, but the op itself went like clockwork.'

'Thank you,' I replied. 'Although it would have been nice to hear that from the surgeon.'

'Oh, don't worry about that,' the guy said, 'he's not so good with families. All that matters is what he does in theatre, right?'

'Yeah,' I said, 'I guess.' But for the first time in my career, I wasn't so sure.

As it turned out, Dad developed renal failure the following day. Nothing to do with the level of skill shown by our errant surgeon – he'd been brilliant, you'd have to say. Not that I could ever tell him that. Never once during the following days did he show his face anywhere near us or even my dad. The anaesthetist, by contrast, was in and out like a nosy neighbour.

My brother was as worried as I was, obviously, but he wouldn't let a word be said about his former boss. An attack on the surgeon was an attack on the whole cardiac family.

'Your lot are just the same,' he insisted. 'Probably worse.'

'You don't know what you're talking about,' I said. 'I've never known a neurosurgeon care so little about his patient or their family.'

He laughed. 'Well, you will, I'm sure of it.'

And, unfortunately, it wasn't long before he was proved right. What this did teach me was about how it feels to be sitting on the cheap sofa, drinking crap coffee and sweating – in other words, being the relative. It was bad enough with my dad as the patient. The amplified terror of it being your baby – you wouldn't want to experience that too often in your life. I knew that part of my job was going to involve trying to manage that fear in other people whenever I could.

Surgery is very much an apprenticeship. You can't learn that much from a book, hence the seemingly never-ending training. At the start, as a junior trainee you spend time examining patients – lots and lots of them – taking care of all the ward work, basically getting to grips with how things are done as much as anything. You're allowed in the operating theatre, but it's a fairly 'no touching' deal. It is a rude demotion compared to the level of operating we did as juniors in other specialities. I was able to do a fair few abdominal procedures almost single-handed, but neurosurgery training puts you right back down again.

After a year of that, you start contributing to some procedures, learning how to close wounds, operating the suction, getting a bit more hands-on. It's very low risk. There's always either a senior trainee or the consultant surgeon – often both – guiding every move. You're nervous as hell the first time you do anything and, though they don't admit it, so are your bosses. But you get through it and the next time they only watch you with one eye.

It was late at night. I was the designated dogsbody on duty, basically there to answer the bleep in case of emergency. But as it turned out, there *was* an emergency and I duly called the senior trainee who was on call with me. He took the patient to theatre. The whole process worked as smoothly as could be hoped. But then the bleep rang again. I took the verbal history and results over the phone from a harassed registrar in some other hospital, no doubt harassed to the extreme also.

I phoned out again to run through the details with my boss, as the senior registrar was busy. Consultants are on call on top of their full-time day duties – so they are at home and are available for advice and assistance. I fully expected him to say, 'Check the patient over – I'm coming in.' But he didn't.

'You've seen this procedure before?' he said.

'Yes.'

'Good, I think you will manage to do this quite fine.'

'Do this? You mean on my own?'

'You want to be a surgeon, don't you?'

'Well, yes, of course.'

'Then he's yours. Let me know how you get on.'

I hung up the phone in shock. At last. It was happening. After all the years of dreaming and waiting, I was finally being allowed to work on my own patient. I was so excited. So ready for my big moment. So determined that this person – this fellow human being – whose life had been placed in my hands, was about to benefit from surely the greatest surgeon the UK would ever see!

I was prepared. I was confident.

Perhaps too confident.

CHAPTER THREE

SEE ONE, DO ONE, TEACH ONE

I'm looking at a patient absolutely riddled with tumours. He has a lymphoma that's spread throughout his body. He's knackered. This is the last roll of the dice. Quite why he has only just appeared on our radar I have no idea. It's clearly been an ongoing problem, but one about to end imminently. I reckon he has no more than twenty-four hours left to live unaided, maybe a few weeks regardless of what we do. Someone would have to operate immediately to give him a fighting chance of having those precious extra days with his family. And that someone, rather unexpectedly, is me.

My boss doesn't seem overly inclined to come in. The senior trainee is already wrists deep in his own surgery. It's time for me to step up.

See one, do one, teach one. The words repeat through my mind. I've seen it, I can do it. It's how it's always been.

I look around and see the anaesthetist who I've worked with before. She looks calm. The scrub nurse has assisted around the operating table for more than twenty years. Just because I'm new, it doesn't mean that there aren't some serious experts in the room.

I've probably seen the operation five times and assisted on it twice. It's fairly straightforward. I need to insert a tube into the man's skull to drain away the excess fluid. The scans show it building up in the ventricles – the fluid spaces we all have in the middle of our brain. If I go in from the patient's right near the front, there's little there of import. All the major speech functions are in the left part of the brain. It's the 'least worst' option, as we are often forced to choose. I've seen and read it many times as being the best entry point.

The patient is covered in green linen drapes. We used to use these for years – washed and reused ad nauseam. Increasing numbers of patches appearing over their lifespan, but only thrown away once they resembled some of my 'battleship-grey' underpants – you know the ones, with extra 'comfort holes' worn in them. Nowadays, it's all disposable. It saves on washing and transport, but I am not sure about the eco-friendliness of all the paper being used. Not my choice any more.

Anyway, I digress. The man's head is partially exposed. Cleaned. Waiting. Ready.

I look to the anaesthetist. 'He's all yours,' she says. 'We're good our end.'

The scrub nurse hands me my scalpel. I make a horseshoe-shape incision around the entry point, then peel back the area of skin. It flaps down, revealing the bone I need to drill through. I look to the scrub nurse. She already has my drill in her hand. She anticipates my every move.

It's crucial not to go too far – to plunge into the brain. Not if you don't want to cause irreparable damage. I set the machine up as I've always seen it done. The power will cut off if I accidentally overstep the distance. It's foolproof.

We're set. We're ready. *Deep breath.*

Anyone who's ever drilled into a plasterboard wall will recognize that familiar lurch when the drill bit breaks through the board and into air. As slowly as I was going, it still came as a shock to suddenly meet no resistance. Except in this case I wasn't drilling air. I'd entered the skull cavity. The drill now off, I opened the fibrous bag around the brain – the dura.

Next, Wendy (the scrub sister) hands me the ventricular drain – the tube I need to pass into the brain to get to the fluid in the middle. Think of it like putting a straw in a coconut to get to the milk inside. I check the markings on the side of the tube as I pass it in: 4 cm; another one to go. I have seen them inserted 5 cm deep before. Now we're in the danger zone. I have to keep moving perfectly forwards. Any deviation could take us away from the fluid and into very sensitive territory. As I read this, it all seems a bit melodramatic. But that's after many years in the job. That initial terror of looking around and realizing there is no cavalry coming – realizing, in fact, that you are the one wearing the fancy blue outfit, coming to save the day. It's hard to forget.

I keep my eyes fixed on the tube's depth markings. It takes less than a second to cover the remaining distance. I can't afford a mistake. A man's life depends on me. I have little experience and all the nerves in the world. It is not his fault that I am the one assigned to saving his life. But it is my privilege. I'm operating on a man's brain. I have the opportunity to save a life, to make a difference. I've dreamed of this moment for so long.

We hit the 5-cm mark and I hear myself sigh with relief. There is a central wire that keeps the tube stiff while I pass it in. I remove it. Fluid starts to come out, and I am utterly relieved. We should see improvements pretty soon.

'We just have to wait till he wakes up,' the anaesthetist says.

I wash up, change out of my scrubs and can barely contain my delight as I leave. If I could have got away with a Fred Astaire-style ankle kick I'd have gone for it. I am buzzing. My first operation. My first test. My first shot at the big time.

Yes, my hands were shaking. All of me was. That wasn't important. What mattered was that I didn't falter during the op. I was Steady Eddie. Cool as a cucumber. Did everything textbook. I was buzzing, on top of the world. Not quite 'God complex' levels but, even if I did say so myself, I'd just tapped into a man's brain – his very soul – and saved his life.

This is what I was born for.

* * ◆ * *

Getting back into the normal swing of things was hard. Apparently, the world hadn't moved on as much as I had.

'Hey, I just performed my first operation.'

'Yay, great – now pass me those suppositories and a sick bowl – this guy's in for a double ender …'

About an hour afterwards, I popped down to the Intensive Care Unit (ICU) to check up on my guy. I was expecting to see my patient upright and chomping on grapes with his loved ones. As it turned out, the mood at the bedside was slightly more sombre. Understandably so.

'When's he going to wake up?' the patient's wife asked. 'When can we take him home?'

What to say? I honestly thought he'd have come round already. 'Well, obviously he's had a serious operation. It went well, but everyone recovers at their own rate. Plus, of course, he was pretty sick from the cancer, so that may mean he will take longer to wake up. But the fluid is draining out, so that should have normalized the pressure in his brain.'

We did overnight on call in addition to the daytime work, so I seamlessly moved from the night emergency cover work into regular daytime stuff. I had a ton of dogsbody chores to plough through for the senior trainee – discharge summaries, referrals back to other hospitals and other low-level work. I dealt with it as best I could, but all the while my mind was in one place: that bed, that man, that operation. That footnote in history.

When my boss announced that he was conducting ward visits, I dumped everything to join in. He hadn't been the one who had been on call and who I'd rung the night before, but I really wanted to show him my proud achievement. For ninety minutes we wandered around the various extremities of the hospital. Finally, we entered ICU. My patient. My reputation.

When the consultant looked at the man's charts he recognized my name. But by then I wasn't particularly paying attention. 'Do you think he should be awake by now?' I asked.

He checked the info. 'Hmm, you would hope so, yes.'

He rattled off questions for the accompanying nurses and his entourage of trainees, and requested further information. He also asked for a new scan. We finished the rest of the round, and then went to look at the scan.

After what seemed like forever, with me standing there fit to burst, he pulled me aside – a generous action as it turned out. 'I don't think he's going to wake up,' he said matter-of-factly, but out of the family's earshot.

'That's not possible,' I spluttered. 'I was the operating surgeon. I did everything right.'

'And yet,' the consultant explained, 'your man is still never going to wake up.'

It was the shittiest moment of my life. I wanted to curl up in a bed alongside my patient and have my own life support switched off.

The patient's scan told a terrible story. Yes, the fluid pressure had been treated, but this had then led to a rapid drop in the pressure of the fluid around the tumour-addled brain. Without that pressure (which was, you will remember, trying in its own evil way to kill the guy), the tumour's blood vessels suddenly felt released and, indeed, released a load of blood into his brainstem – the centre of consciousness and just about everything that keeps you alive. It was a massive bleed. It wasn't my fault and I had had to do the operation. But it didn't stop me feeling incredibly guilty about the whole thing.

'Well, you couldn't have foreseen this, clearly. Seriously, it's not your fault. And in any case,' he added, still staring at the notes, 'he only had days to live anyway. If anything you saved him from a world of suffering.'

◆

I ran up to the neurosurgery floor to find my other boss, the one who had instructed me – and trusted me – to conduct the procedure. As I knocked on the office door I was already writing my speech of resignation. After all, I'd performed an operation which, by the looks of it, was going to shorten a man's life. In other words, the exact opposite of Hippocrates' 'Do no harm' ethos.

I ran through everything I'd done and the horrific outcome. When I finished, the consultant just paused and stroked his chin. 'These things happen,' he said.

'Yes, but it was my fault.'

'It WAS NOT your fault. You did everything right. He was lucky you were there to at least try to save him. His time was up, I'm afraid. Learn from it and move on.'

I was shocked at how forgiving everyone was being.

I left his office, stunned. Relieved, of course, that I hadn't been dragged across the coals. Devastated that the man had died but also confused as to why my bosses didn't seem to be angry. If we were working at a paper-clip factory and I'd mislaid a shipment, then okay, tell me to get over it. But we were surgeons. We were people trusted by the public to save their lives. Surely that should make a difference?

I thought back to my father's case. I remembered how crap we'd all felt being bypassed by the surgeon. It's like we were irrelevant to him. *It really is a God complex,* I thought. *They really think they don't need to answer to anyone.*

With a nauseous gut, and a super supportive senior registrar, I went down to tell the family what had happened. That I had done the operation, but there had been 'unforeseen complications'. It's a peculiarly British method of understatement in the face of a complication that opened the door to death. They listened, thanked me for my honesty and for trying to help. His wife said that he was going to die without the operation and so at least we had given it a go. And that was it.

· · ✦ · ·

The shadow of that operation never went away. I didn't want it to in case I forgot the lessons it had taught me. But life in Wimbledon was too full-on to have that much time to dwell on it. Several of the other consultants went out of their way, I felt, to keep me occupied. I was given handfuls of new cases to prep and consult upon. I really got into the nitty gritty of new patients' requirements, and immersed myself in keeping them and their families up to date right up until the point of surgery.

If I'm honest, I felt like I was being kept busy a bit like a naughty child. Then I realized these other bosses were really just trying to show me that there was always another patient. That I had to be able to cope with these things. Neurosurgery isn't an easy speciality. I needed to learn how to walk the tightrope of caring for my patients, while not becoming paralysed by every complication and knockback. There would be plenty – and some of them could be by my hand. I simply had to learn to accept this and move on, or my career would grind to a halt, with tumours incompletely removed for fear of the consequences and hydrocephalus untreated, plus many other conditions that carried risks dealt with overcautiously. There is a reason that the consent form is chock-full of the potential complications of even the most 'straightforward' brain-surgery operation.

Suck it up, Jayamohan – at least you aren't the patient …

* * ◆ * *

About three weeks after my first solo op, I was due to observe in theatre with a different consultant. The patient looked as though he had a type of tumour called a glioblastoma, something I'd seen a lot of. It was the most malignant type of brain tumour, and almost all of the patients died within nine months to a year, and that was *with* surgery and radiotherapy. I'd 'worked this patient up' – done all the preoperative tests and assessments – and talked to them and really got to know them on the ward, and I guess my boss *du jour* knew this. We were virtually ready to go when she said, 'Look, you've done all the work, do you want to do this op with me? I'll take you through it.'

'Really? I'd love to.'

I never expected to work on a tumour so early in my career. They're the big bad wolves of so much of our work. Being given a chance to operate on it was amazing. The fact I was being trusted to do *anything* after the last time seemed like a miracle. But this boss was incredible. She guided me every step of the way and the operation went like clockwork. The patient woke up and everything was still working for him.

'Not bad at all,' she said afterwards. 'Now, would you like the honour of telling the family?'

'It would be my genuine pleasure. Thank you.'

'A few more dozen of those and maybe – just maybe – you'll be ready to teach one.'

Too soon, boss, too soon …

CHAPTER FOUR

JUST ANOTHER SATURDAY NIGHT

*P*UMP. *PUMP. PUMP.*

The sweat is pouring off me. But it's nothing to the ravines of perspiration seeping down the brow of the anaesthetist. He's the one doing the work. The real work. For now, anyway.

'John,' I shout, 'get in here!'

John is a porter. He lifts, he pushes, he carries all day. He's strong. Fit. Fitter than the anaesthetist. Anaesthetists are some of the most valuable people in a hospital, but you wouldn't want them representing you in a battle. Not when you have porters.

John rushes in. His colleague Dave is behind him. They both know what to do. Taking turns, they pump down on the young man's chest, just as the anaesthetist has been doing. John pumps, he waits, he pumps, he waits. The familiar beads of sweat form on his brow, too. But he can handle it. For now.

PUMP. PUMP. PUMP.

I don't remember the patient's name. All I know for sure is that he's young and he's male. *And he's been dead for three minutes.*

He was alive when he came in. Just. His pupils were dilated and his head showed signs of massive trauma. He'd been beaten to a pulp outside a pub an hour earlier – *just another Saturday night.* A scan in A&E had identified a blood clot on the brain and so they'd shipped him across to me. They didn't hold out much hope, but even as they handed over the trolley one of them said, 'Hope you've got your miracle-worker shoes on for this one.'

It's a running joke. Everyone knows that neurosurgeons believe themselves to be the top of the medical tree. That's what we like to tell ourselves – and anyone else who'll listen. No one believes it, until you get a mashed-up mess like this and then it's time to try to live up to the myth.

PUMP. PUMP. PUMP.

The patient's heart stopped the second we got him on the operating table. 'Oh, *bugger.*'

Everyone thought or said the same thing as the heart monitor ceased beeping and hit that all-too-familiar continuous eerie note. But it was the anaesthetist who said it loudest. The heart's his domain in theatre. I might be the one with the magic knife, but he's in charge of keeping the patient breathing till I'm done. Whichever way you look at it, a 'flatliner' doesn't sit well on anyone's scorecard.

Before anyone else had reacted, he'd gone straight into chest compression mode with his hands. Electric paddles can sometimes jump-start a heart, but that takes time to set up, and there were enough bits of metal equipment around the patient to electrocute a few of us in the process.

So, manual stimulation it was. It's nothing like what you see in the movies. Unless you're close to breaking the patient's ribs, you're not doing it right. And pressing hard enough to do that, again and again and again, is exhausting. Hence the call to the boys.

PUMP. PUMP. PUMP.

'Four minutes, Jay,' the anaesthetist says, just about keeping it together.

Four minutes? The guy's been gone longer than it takes some people to run a mile. When, I wonder, does a person turn from a patient into a corpse? It's odd the things you think about in such moments.

After what seems like an interminable amount of time, we get a pulse, and a blood pressure, of sorts. The patient was still super rickety and could go down again at any time. We discuss what to do. Ideally, we would want to spend some time getting him on various medicines in the ITU – the intensive care unit – to support his heart. But it had stopped because of the blood clot in his beaten-up brain – without me getting the clot out, he was a goner anyway. So, we decide that I will operate and they will keep his heart going with medicines and hands, depending on how it goes.

There are two ways to open a person's head. The pretty way and the quick way. Usually, I shave the hair, use a scalpel to nick the skin, then apply an electrocautery device to burn down to bone level. It's a slow, precise method and it leaves almost no scarring. But it takes time. Time, the incessant beeping note of the heart monitor reminds me, I don't have. The fastest way is the only option.

'For God's sake, Jay, get him open, get the clot. Let's go, go, go!'

I don't need to be told, but again the anaesthetist is only saying what everyone else is thinking. I plant the knife blade against the man's skin and press down. It goes deep and I feel it connect with the bone. I make the incision in the shape of a question mark. I drag back the skin and muscle, and I stare at the bone. It wasn't a neat-looking procedure, but was the quickest way in. If I don't do something now, there is no future. Not for this guy.

Five minutes have gone by.

It's in an emergency like this that you appreciate the value of a great scrub nurse. The good ones know what I need before I do. The really good ones have it ready as soon as I put out my hand. But the great ones place the tool in my hand exactly how I want it, so I don't need to take my eyes from the patient for a second. Jill is one of the best. She hands me the drill.

'What's taking so long?'

More cheerleading from the anaesthetist. I love the night-shift team spirit. It's more like squabbling siblings – we bitch at each other, but always have each other's backs.

The drill is calibrated to puncture the skull then cut out before it damages the brain. It's just as well, the speed I'm hammering the first hole. One down, two to go. Again and again I lean into the device, wincing instinctively as the fine shards of bone spiral into the ether.

Two. Three. Now it's time to join the dots.

'Six minutes.'

Jill plants the jigsaw into my outstretched palm, trigger perfectly aligned to my forefinger and thumb. I clutch the saw, insert the thin blade inside one of the holes and power up. It's hard work. Being up against the clock makes everything tougher, every tool heavier. But I lean into the angle and feel my hand dip slightly as the first connection is made.

The next two lines take another minute or so. As I drag the blade across for the final time, I'm aware of the fear in the room being replaced by a palpable tension. We're nearly there. Make or break time.

'Eight minutes, Jay. Hurry up, for Christ's sake.'

I nod imperceptibly. It's all that's required. He knows I've heard. He also knows I don't need to be told. But he's a solid guy. Sometime before, I had moved up to Glasgow to further my training, we have both been registrars there for a couple of years, and have done many a night on call together. We trust each other, and that's worth more than anything in this situation.

If I've done my sums right, the bleeding clot shutting down the messages to the heart – and everything else – should be directly underneath the rough pentagon shape I'm carving out. Given the circumstances, I've made the hole bigger than usual. At small palm size, I should be able to find what I'm looking for below. I'm as anxious as anyone to get there.

The scrub nurse takes the saw almost before I hold it out to her. Seconds later, my fingers are prising out the five-sided island I've cut out of bone. Now it's my turn to sweat.

'Come on, come on …'

My fingers seem to swell with every passing second, but suddenly I make contact and the jagged piece of skull lifts clean off in my hand. The dura is roughly sliced open with a knife, then cut with big scissors – no time for mucking about here. Below it, I should see a brain. In its place, all I can make out is a bloody lump covered in what appears to be jam. It's the clot, and it's massive.

The anaesthetist is shouting now, desperate. But his voice is not what I'm listening to. I'm ignoring the porters' exhausted grunts, too. What's grabbing my attention isn't in fact a noise at all. It's the absence of one. The lack. Is it my imagination or has the piercing repetitive noise of the heart monitor stopped?

The anaesthetist suddenly notices, too. 'Come on, you bastard.'

We all know what should happen next, but the wait is excruciating.

Then it comes, faintly at first. *Beep. Beep.*

Then stronger. *BEEP. BEEP. BEEP. BEEP.*

I smile. I can't help it. The act of removing a portion of the skull has been sufficient to alleviate the pressure on the brain. Communication channels to the heart and lungs are restored. As is normal service among my colleagues.

I keep working as the patient stabilizes. There's still work to be done. I need to suction out the blood and remove any damaged brain that is too far gone to ever work again. Then I plate the skull back together and replace the patient's skin as neatly as I can. But we've done it. We've achieved the impossible. We've brought a man back from the dead. Interfered with the natural order of things and turned a corpse back into a patient.

I smile again as I rejoin the skull. I realize that this is what I want to do forever.

Just another Saturday night in Glasgow …

· · ◆ · ·

You never stop learning. When you're a junior, you basically operate all the time because you work for several bosses, and as soon as you're free you just operate on the next patient. That's why within six years you go from not being able to pick up a knife, to becoming a consultant. At least, that's the dream. It's a very intense process. I had two years at Ealing and Wimbledon as a junior surgeon, then known as the 'Senior House Officer'. I was notching up many, many more operations – increasingly unsupervised and much more rewarding. They were of differing specialities, but all increased my skills.

The goal was to reach the level of neurosurgical registrar. To my mind those were – and are – the guys who run the hospital. You're with the patients all the time. You live on the ward. You know everything about everyone coming in. Some consultants will rely entirely on your notes when they conduct their assessments. Some will get more involved and press the flesh with the families and the patients. But, as I already knew to my cost, all that touchy-feely stuff was purely optional for the *grands fromages* with the scalpels. So it's the registrar who is essential to the process. I couldn't have been looking forward to it more.

As competition was super stiff I followed the work. I didn't have a PhD, which put me at a distinct disadvantage when it came to applying for jobs. Nineteen forms went in with no interview. I had become so disillusioned with my chances to the point where I had wondered about other options, like retraining to become a barrister. I didn't want to end up a bitter doctor doing a job I didn't like. Plus, I have a penchant for arguing. It stood me in good stead in the years ahead, but more of that later.

Then Glasgow had a vacancy for a registrar in neurosurgery, so I went for it and was invited to come up. The interview was totally different compared to filling in forms. I could put forward my argument about why I hadn't taken three years out to do research. I didn't know which sub-speciality to devote my career to, so I would just be doing what the academics told me to do. But I didn't want that – I wanted to treat patients. I wanted to cut, to help them get better, just as I did all those years ago as a student in London. They actually understood that view and, at long last, with almost the last roll of the dice, I got the job. I sold my flat in London and I headed up to stay there for the next five years.

I discovered just what an amazing city it was. Bars, restaurants, clubs and a population that knew how to party. It was fun central – and the guys at work were simply fantastic. From top to bottom, we really were a family. But I also realized that, sometimes, Glasgow was driven by more negative emotions.

For those unaware of the city's sporting history, there are two football behemoths fighting each other for supremacy. And when I say fighting, I do mean it literally. Like so many places in the world, religion is at the heart of the divide. Glasgow Rangers are, historically, linked with the Protestant faith, whereas their counterparts Glasgow Celtic are predominantly Catholic in fan base. It shouldn't matter. Faith is about positivity and love. Football is about escapism and fitness – messages that sometimes don't seem to have filtered through to Scotland's second city.

Each football match between the two clubs – known as an 'Old Firm derby' – has the police on overtime. If sporting rivalry doesn't kick off a riot then sectarianism is waiting in the wings. Basically, you're always just a conversation away from a bloodbath. Or, as stupid as it may sound, the wrong colour car can land you in hot water.

On my first day in Glasgow, I arrived full of the joys of spring. My first shift was perfectly fine. I left late and happened to walk down to the car park with one of the other senior trainees. We were still chatting as I stopped outside my trusty old blue Honda.

'Is this yours?' he asked.

'Yeah. It's no Aston Martin, but it gets me from A to B.'

'It'll get you to A&E if you're not careful.'

'What are you talking about?'

'Seriously? It's blue. It's the colour of Rangers. Approximately half the city is going to want to smash it.'

'Don't be ridiculous. My shirt's blue as well. Am I in danger because of that?'

'It depends where you go.'

It was hyperbole, of course, but not as far from reality as you might think. The young man who we'd brought back from the dead on the operating table was a case in point. Attacked for being in the wrong football shirt in the wrong part of town. Pathetic, really. But some people weren't even safe at home.

Glasgow has its fair share of tenement buildings and, because of its weather, few air-conditioning units. One hot summer Sunday, a bunch of 'fans' were watching the Old Firm match on TV with the front door open. The game had just finished – not in their team's favour – when one of them saw a flash of colour pass by on the landing.

'Get him,' he said, and ran for the doorway. His mates weren't slow in following. In the stairwell they found a young man wearing the familiar strip of their mortal enemy and, because they were morons, they just leapt on him. One of them ran back to the flat and returned with hammers, bats and a golf club. They really went to town on the poor sod. And all because of his fashion choice that morning.

By the time I laid eyes on him, he was barely recognizable as a man. The CT scan revealed a massive brain injury. It also gave some clues as to the cause. I could make out individual dents in the skull that looked remarkably like hammer marks and at least one made by a five iron.

'The weapon of the coward,' my boss said. 'A lot of these toerags carry golf clubs as weapons because if police stop them they say they're going to the driving range. Get used to it.'

He was pretty much dead on the table before we'd got moving. But we had a go at operating because he was young. No life should be more valuable than another's, but this young man had so much more to live for. And the way he'd died was just so … *avoidable*.

There was a room next to the theatre where the lad's family were waiting. My boss saw me wavering outside the door. She could tell I was really stressing out – it was the first patient I'd attended to who had died on account of the colour of his shirt. I couldn't get my head around it.

'I'll tell them if you want,' she said. 'No one will judge you.'

'I'll judge me,' I said. 'I want to do this.'

Inside were people whose son, uncle or brother had died needlessly. As the surgeon in charge of the operation, I felt it was my responsibility – my duty – to impart the news.

I thought long and hard about what I was going to say. In cases like that you have to be prepared for them to turn on you. 'Why didn't you save him?' You see it all and you can't blame them. But it turned out words were unnecessary. The second I walked through the door, the mum burst into tears. She could read it on my face.

'Not my bairn. Not my wee bairn!'

It was heartbreaking. I sat with them to go through the events of the day in detail, but really no one was listening. When I finished, the young man's brother shook my hand.

'Thank you for trying,' he said. 'It means everything.'

* * ◆ * *

Sometimes it wasn't the colour of your clothes that got you in trouble. It wasn't even your choice of car. It was your skin.

A guy was admitted after having been thumped around and had suffered significant head injuries. Casualty had given him the once-over and they'd sent him to us. He had an open wound to his head that needed surgery, as well as a fractured cheekbone. He was a total charmer. The moment I walked into the room, he said to the nurse, 'I don't want that Paki operating on me.' Even his broken face wasn't enough to stop him from spitting his venom.

She didn't bat an eyelid. 'Well, since he's the only surgeon here, you've got a choice: him or death.' Sure, not strictly true on any of those points, but she was pretty cheesed off, and I wasn't going to correct her.

I thought that once we got him unconscious that would be the end of it. In fact, he was more angry and vile when naked than when he was awake. Every inch of his torso was inked with Nazi imagery or propaganda. I've never seen so many swastikas in one place. Of course, he wasn't all bad. To prove his softer side, he had the words 'All for you' tattooed above his groin with a downwards arrow pointed at his knob. A lovely chap.

I managed to clean his head injury and suture it up, and my maxillofacial surgeon colleague rebuilt the mashed bones so he no longer had 'a face like a melted welly' as they say in Scotland. We couldn't have done more. Likewise, his wife couldn't have been more grateful.

'I apologize for him being such an arse,' she said. 'I can't do anything about it.'

I don't just hang around to deliver bad news, so I wanted to tell the guy that he was, in all likelihood, going to make a near-perfect recovery and be back on his racist feet in no time. Which I did.

I wondered how long he could hold his tongue … About ten seconds, as it transpired.

'Get the fuck off me,' he yelled. 'I don't want you lot touching me.'

'My lot? You mean neurosurgeons?'

'I mean Pakis.'

'No Pakis here. I'm from Sri Lanka.'

The nurse laughed. His wife said something ineffectual. He twitched like he'd been electrocuted.

'Oh, I wasn't the only one who touched you,' I said. 'I'd like to introduce you to the person who reconstructed your beautiful face,' – and I beckoned in my colleague who, for maximum effect, made sure his Star of David necklace hung prominently over his smock. 'And of course you've met your nurse?' Netty, the most amazing Jamaican angel, blew him a kiss.

The fury on his face. I could still hear him swearing as I reached the end of the corridor.

We took solace from the fact that the so-called 'master race' disciple required help from black, white and all colours in between to wipe his nose, drain his pee from the catheter and wipe his bum. But it soon wore thin. I think I hoped he'd see the error of his ways. That he'd come to acknowledge that without the very people he detested, he'd possibly be six-foot underground. No such luck. He hated us with as much venom from day one until discharge. We got to the stage where he'd pretend to be asleep rather than watch a 'foreigner' touch his body.

'I suppose we could go back in and cut out the racist part?' my colleague said to me, with a wink, one day when we were in our office. 'Perhaps,' he said, 'you could make him love brownies.'

Even a specialism like neurosurgery has sub-specialisms and, by the time I finished at Glasgow, I'd be expected to focus on one. The only problem was, I loved the lot. Every single aspect. As with junior doctor training, you get moved on rotation from one specialist department to another, from spinal surgery to epilepsy surgery to tumour surgery to trauma surgery, all the big guns and various others. Within days of seeing each new set-up I'd think, *This is amazing. This is what I want to specialize in. This is what I*

want to spend the rest of my life doing. Then six months later I'd be somewhere else and change my mind entirely. And so it went on until I reached neurosurgical paediatrics.

There was an instant connect, and for several reasons – some more altruistic than others. The first thing I noticed about the department was how they really kept the family involved in every decision. Whatever the children were in for, the consultant did his or her best to make sure the family were up to speed. It was such a pleasure to see this after some of the shoddy pastoral care I'd experienced in London. So why was I still not happy?

You can be a bit of cock when you're a registrar, thinking you could do better than your boss. I was, and I did. It took me no time at all to realize that some of the consultants weren't just talking to the family – they were *only* talking to the family. What about little Nancy or Kevin tucked up in bed? The kids were the real patients – so why were they being ignored?

Full disclosure: I think I've always had a healthy relationship with my inner child. Possibly too healthy. I love video games, PlayStation, reading comics like *2000AD* and *Calvin and Hobbes*, and almost any cartoons. I love slapstick humour, I love *The Simpsons*. Yes, I'm basically immature. But you know who else are? Kids.

You can sometimes see adults talk to children in a smarmy politician 'Hey, kids. What's happening?' sort of style and it smacks of fakery. Kids know when they're being spoken down to. They really don't go for that. They are very good at sensing when an adult is trying too hard to be their friend and just think, *I don't really know what you're doing or what you think you're doing, but you're not fooling me in any way, shape or form.* Fortunately, I realized that I could relate to my tinier patients very easily and talk to them on a level they could identify with. I wouldn't say it's a skill, more just me. I felt I knew what they needed. And what they needed, more than anything, was some level of honesty.

If you're the one lying in bed with drips coming out of your arm and a pain in your head that you can't scratch, you're going to be terrified. Imagine watching Mum and Dad huddle in a corner, whispering to a stranger in a white coat (we still wore them for lots of my training). You know they're talking about you. What are they saying? Am I going to die?

Of course, if you don't talk to that child and explain to them what's going on, their imagination will kick into overdrive and what they come up with will probably be double or triple as serious as what's actually going on. Kids aren't stupid. They know when something's wrong. They know that there's something not quite right with them. They're in a hospital, for Pete's sake. You need to be able to explain the situation to them to ensure they feel comfortable and understand what's going on in a way they can process. What you mustn't do is treat them like they're invisible, which some of my colleagues appeared more comfortable doing. To be honest, so did some parents. They occasionally hated it when we were honest with their child. They thought they were protecting them by withholding the truth. There were fraught times, but my consultants always had my back.

With my time at Glasgow coming to an end, I needed to make a choice. There was only one real candidate. I realized I had a level of attachment to paediatrics that went above anything I felt for the other departments. I honestly believed I could do some serious good in that world.

But, if I'm honest, that wasn't the only reason I elected to go down that path. In my time in paediatrics I saw myriad different cases, watched consultants scratching their heads, and then got to open up the hood of babies and 6-foot teenagers. No two cases were the same. And it was thrilling. I pictured a life specializing in adult spine surgery. Yes, practice makes perfect. Yes, after a while I could become the go-to guy in the field. I could become the top man in the industry. But, oh my God, the tedium. The prospect of being pigeon-holed in one tiny aspect of my training. The idea of doing the same thing every single day crushed me. Whereas with kids, you never knew what you were going to find.

Decision made, there was only one place I wanted to go. I booked a flight to Canada.

* * ◆ * *

Known as 'SickKids', the Hospital for Sick Children in Toronto takes patients from a huge swathe of Canada, numbering about nine million people. If I was going to get up to speed on paediatric neurosurgery, it seemed the perfect place to go. It had to be – I was gambling a lot on it working.

At the time, my then fiancée was doing a research degree in Glasgow, so she couldn't travel. We couldn't sell my flat because she needed somewhere to live. So I took a pretty hefty loan from Barclays and packed my bags. Spoiler alert: it was totally worth it and probably the best investment I have ever made (other than marrying my fiancée!).

I arrived as a 'Fellow', ostensibly to work alongside more highly trained seniors and consultants and learn from them. Mostly it worked out that way.

The set-up at SickKids was fantastic. As you can imagine, covering the entire east coast there was a lot of opportunity for daily operating as everyone was kept very busy. The consultants were among the world's most well-respected experts, comprising academics as well as clinicians. I wasn't the only visiting Fellow. They get people from all over the world coming to work for them basically for free (I had been awarded a £500 per month scholarship to help towards rent), just because it's *the* place to go and train. Even the juniors, like me, are actually very experienced by the time they arrive at the end of their training, so the whole environment is on another level. I'd have paid to work there.

Lots of the work that came in was tumour-related. You can never work too many tumour cases. Certainly never relax. The risk of devastating failure is always a hair's breadth away. You need a very specific knowledge of 3D anatomy, excellent hand-eye coordination – what is often called a 'visuospatial skill subset' – which I, like everyone else there, was trying to learn at breakneck speed. Even so, every operation I performed, either as lead surgeon with supervision or helping a consultant, was a challenge. Albeit a very rewarding challenge.

Outside theatre I found dealing with Canadian kids and parents just as straightforward as in the UK. I knew I was on to something. I knew I could make a difference back home. As it turned out, I soon made a difference in Toronto.

You don't automatically become a 'consultant' – there's a formal job application and interview process. Once successful, you finish your last training day and then essentially move offices and get a new shiny ID badge. But going from registrar on a Monday to consultant on a Tuesday doesn't necessarily imbue you with any more experience. I worked with a couple of bosses who were barely a year older than me. One had literally returned from his year's fellowship the day before I arrived and now he was suddenly expected to step up to the top level. It's all about how you handle it and he handled it brilliantly. They all had great attitudes, totally inclusive in the way they worked, always asking questions of their juniors. Not a 'see one, do one, teach one' in sight.

I learned a phrase from one of them that I have stolen for myself. Jim would say, 'Now, if you see me doing something stupid, for f***'s sake please say something straightaway. Don't wait for me to screw up. You're my backup.' This, coming from one of the most experienced paediatric neurosurgeons in the world to a baby like me, was a really brilliant attitude that I try to emulate.

One day a head trauma came in and the senior surgeon asked for comments. I'd seen and worked on tens of trauma cases in Glasgow.

It was basically the bread and butter of the department. So I was full of suggestions.

'Perhaps you'd like to lead on this one, Jay?' he said.

And with echoes of a previous professional exchange, once again I replied, 'It would be my pleasure.'

It says a lot for the cultural differences, I suppose, that I, a relatively junior import from Glasgow, had significantly more trauma experience than the home-grown consultant in Toronto. But I'm not one to look a gift horse in the mouth and absolutely relished the extra responsibility whenever one of these terrible cases came in.

And they *were* terrible, because of course not all trauma cases are accidental. In fact, in my experience in adult neurosurgery, they were quite often not accidents at all.

Ah yes, but that was in Glasgow, I thought, as I looked at the scan of my new patient's battered brain. *That was with stupid, drunken, blinkered men. This is a six-month-old baby. No one would do that intentionally.*

I glanced at the parents. *Or would they?*

CHAPTER FIVE

BATMAN AND ROBIN

The three underpinnings of any sort of diagnosis are: take a history, examine the patient, do some tests. Occasionally, the history and the investigation can completely fight against each other.

A baby was brought in one day with head trauma. A couple of trainees had passed on it as they preferred the tumours. I was next in line. The child was unwell, clearly. The problem I had wasn't with the injury, but the parents. The story changed half-hourly.

'She fell.'

'This basket toppled on her.'

'The dog pushed her over.'

'She was hiding under a table and looked up too quickly.'

Some of the explanations you could rule out by age alone. Baby was eight months old. She can't walk, so she's not falling. Dog knocked her over? It would have had to pick her up first. The others were suspicious simply because of the many other stories. I was convinced something had happened that the family wasn't telling us about.

These two people were allegedly with the child throughout and yet they couldn't say what had happened. Even they had to see how bad that looked. But they didn't.

Usually people come in saying, 'Little Johnny's been vomiting, gone off his feet, he's wobbly, his arm is twitching' – something that gives us an idea of where to start looking. We do the investigation, we find the abnormalities, we treat. Things progress in a fairly predictable manner. Throw in the extra variable of wondering whether people are telling the truth or not and everything becomes very unpredictable indeed.

At thirty-three, I was at the stage where I knew I was going to qualify as a paediatric neurosurgeon and I would be looking for a job within the year. You have a little bit of a swagger at this time. Perhaps some overconfidence about what you know. You've dedicated your whole life and a lot of money to get to where you are – and I don't just mean Canada. It comes with the territory that you're so certain about things.

And I was certain that this family was lying. Absolutely. Cast-iron guarantee. Interrogating them, however, wasn't my job. Not my real job. My duty was to ascertain the nature of the injury and treat it as quickly and effectively as possible. I could report the parents to the social services once the child was safe.

The injury was, I thought at the time, a very classic trauma event. I couldn't work out what else it could be. I operated, removing the swelling in the brain by drilling into the skull. Two hours in and out. As I stitched her up, I questioned the point of it all. Was I just patching the child up so she could be abused another day? Maybe. Maybe not.

One of my colleagues found me afterwards. 'We've got the investigation results,' she said, waving a batch of papers. 'It turns out Baby has a bleeding disorder.'

'Let me see that.' I scanned through the notes and there in black and white was the bald fact that this child had a propensity to bleed with far less cause than was common for most people. So this could explain the condition, the bleeding within the skull causing brain dysfunction, but not the dodgy behaviour of the parents.

'You know something's really fishy about them, don't you?' I said.

'Sure do.'

'Why would they be like that if they're innocent?'

She shrugged.

The whole episode made me pull up short. I'd been so confident of one scenario having played out, but in all likelihood there was an alternative explanation. I didn't want to make the same mistake again. Jumping to conclusions helps nobody, least of all the patient.

I began reading as much around the subject as I could. A pathologist called Dr John Plunkett wrote an article in *The British Medical Journal* about child abuses. Plunkett is somebody who does not believe in shaken baby syndrome. He doesn't accept that you can shake a baby to death without causing profound neck injury, and supplied page after page of reasoned argument and evidence. It was certainly food for thought.

I'd been educated to believe that facts were immutable. Medical school is full of facts – we learnt them and put them into practice. Easy-peasy it seemed to us, in our innocence (or naivety, depending on your view). Now, it seemed, they were only part of a puzzle. Context had to be considered as well. It wasn't long, however, before I realized that even this could be manipulated.

I left Canada a few months later, never really knowing whether my patient's flaky parents had something to hide or not. I was taking up a neurosurgical post at the John Radcliffe Hospital in Oxford. More importantly, at the age of thirty-four, I had finally achieved my goal of becoming a consultant.

But if Canada had taught me anything, it is that you never stop learning. I was a consultant, but a junior one. Ahead of me was my mentor and, very quickly, my friend Peter Richards. Peter was a great senior person to have around. He'd been there, done that, got the T-shirt, worn it out and bought another one. By coincidence he also was – *is* – one of the UK's most experienced neurosurgeons, looking at cases of alleged child abuse in the legal field. When he learned I had a burgeoning interest in that side of things he said, 'If you want to look at some of my cases, let me know.'

'I'd like that.'

'But I warn you: it's not a world to enter lightly.'

I soon discovered what he meant. I was referred by Peter to offer advice in a case where a two-year-old had died of trauma to the head. There was video evidence of the mother's boyfriend repeatedly hitting the child. He actually recorded himself. It took me several attempts to finish each clip. I'm a surgeon, I'm not squeamish and I'm certainly not afraid of blood. But I do what I do because I want to heal. To fix. Having to watch and listen to this criminal savagery was harrowing.

The jury certainly thought so. There was silence in the courtroom as the videos were played. You could hear a pin drop. The only sounds were the agonizing screams of the poor little mite – and the occasional gasp and retching noise as jurors' stomachs turned.

Undoubtedly, the boyfriend was an animal. Clearly, he had subjected an innocent child to unimaginable pain for the entirety of its short life. But – the defence team wanted to know – was he responsible for the baby's death? And that is where things got tricky.

There was overwhelming evidence to indicate that the man was a monster. A child abuser. A bully. There was no doubt he had caused injury upon injury. But, his barrister asked, 'Can you, in your expert opinion, honestly say that you see a fatal blow being delivered?'

As much as I wanted to say yes, I had to be honest. 'No.'

'Can you say, definitively, that the defendant is the only person to have struck the child?'

Well, who else? I thought. But again the answer was, 'No.'

'Could it, possibly, have been the child's mother who delivered the fatal blow? Or someone else?'

And then it became clear. The defence's argument wasn't that the boyfriend hadn't abused the child – that was all caught on tape, there was no denying it. Rather it was that he couldn't be proven to have murdered him. *They were going for reasonable doubt.*

However, it didn't work. The defendant was found guilty of murder by a sickened jury. But I left the court with more questions than answers. For all my great leaps forward in Toronto, learning not to judge a book by its cover, I had to face a new realization: that even facts and accuracy and truth can be distorted if you squint hard enough.

· · ◆ · ·

Work on legal cases had to be squeezed in around clinical work. Before I joined, Peter's department was just him. My arrival doubled the consultant staff and the workload. In the early days we'd do the ward rounds together, so he could get me up to speed. We were inseparable. Maybe a bit too inseparable.

'You know what the nurses are calling us?' he said, one day.

'Nothing good, I imagine.'

'Batman and Robin.'

'That's not so bad,' I said. 'But which one of us is Batman?'

He burst out laughing. 'I don't know, Robin. You tell me.'

· · ◆ · ·

The John Radcliffe Hospital's very own Bruce Wayne was pretty old school in a lot of ways, but he didn't have the ego that, in my experience, often went with it. Along with the ridiculous workload, he was happy to share the credit. More importantly, when stumped, he wouldn't just go with our joint best guess for the sake of looking clever.

Case in point: I had a child with a difficult vascular malformation, a lesion on the brain. I say 'I' because Peter let me take every case that I wanted. He was in a position in his life where he didn't need to take on any more cases to build up experience, so it worked really well. Of course, the fact that you've just become a consultant doesn't mean suddenly you know everything. You're the same chump that you were the day before, when you were the senior registrar. The first years (or even the first decade) as a consultant can then be spent building up a large list of cases. Doctors have a great ability to remember things, but now, as consultants, we can get rid of the 'stupid', rare diseases we had to learn about as students and would never see, and fill the memory banks with relevant, well-indexed experience – the stuff with which we could go into battle against the diseases and conditions encountered in whichever specialism we had chosen.

The type of vascular malformation in front of me now wasn't anything I'd encountered before, so naturally I asked Peter. Not surprisingly, he had seen it and dealt with it before but, because it was so rare in kids, not for a very long time. 'I can check my notes,' he said.

'What about if I ask my old bosses in Toronto?' I asked. 'I know one of them has got a particular interest in this area.'

The idea of asking an outside source – and a foreign one at that – for help would be enough to ruin some of the 'old school' people I'd trained with. But not Peter. 'Splendid idea. Let me know what they say. Quite probably things have moved on since I last treated it anyway.'

I fired off an email to Toronto and thus began a series of transatlantic ping-pong as ideas flew back and forth between us. I told them my observations and my planned line of attack, and they, very gently, told me better alternatives. They never said: 'Don't do that, you idiot.' It was more: 'Have you considered …?' or 'Ever think about this approach?'

It was a really collegiate atmosphere, very respectful and, in the long term, exceptionally influential. It's how I swore I would always try to treat anyone who ever had the misfortune in the future to work for me. It doesn't always work because there are some people who are too uncaring or lazy to have become doctors in the first place – something that drives me bonkers as a teacher.

The long and short of it was that everyone in the loop agreed on one idea, so I took it to Peter.

'That sounds like a great plan. Let's do that,' he confirmed.

We did and it worked. Even if it hadn't, it was still the best way forward. Like I said, you never stop learning. You never stop wanting to improve. You never stop wanting to help.

Sometimes, though, that isn't enough. In fact, sometimes those instincts can cause more problems than they solve. As I was about to find out.

CHAPTER SIX

THAT'S NOT FAT

Eight months. It's no age. No age to die. No age to be born. Not like this.

Not even eight months old. This is eight months BC – Before Caesarean. Before Coming into this world. It's tragic.

The baby had popped up on my radar antenatally, after Mum complained of not feeling any kicks or movements or any of those other things that pregnant women can sense and enjoy. Her local hospital did a scan of the foetus. Often it turns out to be something that's fixable. That's what they were looking for. In this instance they found that Baby had a brain tumour.

Breaking that news to the parents of a five-year-old is hard enough. But telling expectant parents that the unborn child they haven't even met yet might have a terminal disease is crushing.

'A tumour?' Mum says, her face white in shock. Her husband clutches her hand. It won't help either of them to learn that the condition is relatively rare. That there were just over 400 brain tumours in under-eighteen-year-olds in 2018 – in the UK. Maybe this was the only baby to be diagnosed at this stage in the whole country. It's all irrelevant to them.

Dad looks at his wife, his hand drifts to her tummy. He looks at me, then back to them. 'Oh my God,' he says, 'our baby's got cancer.'

· · ◆ · ·

You can't blame him. When people hear the word 'tumour' they automatically think of the 'Big C'. It's understandable, but not what the word means.

A tumour is a lump. An area of tissue that has experienced accelerated growth. If the tumour is the sort that tends to stay in the same location and slowly gets bigger within the same place, and just pushes the brain out of the way, that tends to be what we call benign. As opposed to the tumours which can move around the bloodstream or the cerebrospinal fluid between the brain and the spinal cord. These tumours have the ability to detach a portion of themselves off, float off, reattach in various locations and start to grow there as well. Those are what we call cancer cells.

There are lots and lots of different types of cells that work together to form the brain. It's not all just nerve cells. These are very delicate and require an elaborate scaffolding of supporting – or glial – cells to give them the ability to make the connection with each other. There are supporting cells and insulating cells, cells that are there to supply energy and oxygen, and cells that the neurons themselves hang onto.

The texture and the appearance of a tumour will very much depend on which cell type it comes from. Tumours in the nerve cells are actually relatively rare. The most common are tumours of the glial cells – they make the scaffolding for the nerves. These are cells which tend to replicate and grow over time, replacing each other. In most people it all goes to plan. Occasionally, the cells replicate but misread the recipe book, forget to add an 'off switch' and just keep growing into what becomes a tumour.

With neonatal cases there's an added layer of confusion. At that age cells are still in a state of flux, they're literally growing right in front of you. What you have to ask yourself is: are you looking at rapidly growing cancer cells or just cells that are growing because they're still supposed to be *in utero*? There's much we still don't understand.

MRI scans revolutionized medical treatment. In the case of tumours, however, they can only do so much. You can't tell a malignant tumour from a benign one just by looking. A tumour comprising 10 per cent of the brain can prove more toxic than one covering 20 per cent. Or, in this instance, 50 per cent. Whether they're highly malignant or benign, there's no way of knowing at first glance. Bottom line: they all look bad till you get inside.

Still, there are always options.

The later you leave a termination, the harsher it is for the carrier. You can dress it up however you like, but basically the medical team will often end the baby's life, with the mother still needing to deliver the body. I can't think of a much more traumatic scenario than a mother having to give birth to a child whose medical condition was so serious, she agreed to terminate their life. There's no hearing the first cry, there's no first feed. It's unimaginably distressing. But sometimes it's the way that parents choose to go.

This baby was just past eight months of development when her condition was flagged. Way past the 'normal' dates when mothers decide to have an abortion. But these conditions were anything but normal. In situations where birth can be injurious to the health of the mother, or a baby is really sick, then termination remains an option throughout pregnancy.

But the mother needs to decide. Although fathers are often involved in such a momentous decision, legally it is only the mother who can make the final call either way.

Baby's mum hears the evidence, takes in the severity of her unborn child's condition, understands the real likelihood of her baby dying, if not in childbirth then shortly after. She hears it all and, after discussion with her husband, decides to press ahead with the pregnancy anyway.

I'm there at the birth, a month after the dreadful news had been broken. The mother had to go through that four weeks in constant stress and anxiety – every time she couldn't feel the baby move, she must have been so worried.

Scans can only tell you so much. I need to see with my own eyes what I will be dealing with later. Will I have to operate tonight or do I have a couple of weeks to prep the case properly and study the baby?

We recommended a birth by Caesarean section as we weren't really sure how Baby's head would cope with the pressure of standard delivery. Her tumour accounted for a significant part of the brain mass and there were too many variables to risk.

The birth goes well and Baby emerges breathing and functioning as you would hope. No way had that been a given. Such a large tumour could easily have pressed hard enough on the brain to block vital passageways. On top of that, the pressure outside the womb is different to inside. There was no telling how she was going to react physically, but not only is she functioning, she is thriving. Watching Mum hold her, you would have no idea there was a problem.

But we both knew there was. From my point of view, I could see I had time to fully explore what had to be done. To get blood cross-matched for a transfusion, to do MRI scans, to really get a sense of what we were dealing with.

If things hadn't gone to plan, we weren't exactly on DEFCON 1 but we were prepared. We would have had theatre ready within the day. We could have drained any fluid build-up inside the head, any number of things. It isn't necessary. Even so, Baby is sent to SCBU – Special Care Baby Unit – while I request the MRI.

◆

Tumours appear for different reasons. First guess historically has always been genetics. Our tests found no obvious cause in either parent's lineage. These days there is a whole area called epigenetics, which studies the way that the environment changes your genes, even *in utero*. It's interesting stuff, but not particularly helpful when you're staring at a tumour that's only going to keep growing.

Despite their bad press, it can be malignant brain tumours that pose a lesser threat than their 'benign' cousins. Or, at least, a more treatable one. Due to their cells' rapid replication, they often prove susceptible to chemotherapy and can be treated without invasive surgery, just a biopsy. I know I'm a surgeon, but I'm never happier than if I *don't* have to operate at all on a newborn. There's always someone else who *does* need an operation.

Tumours in the brain differ from elsewhere in the body. Or, more accurately, our responses to them do. At face value, people think that having a malignant tumour must be terrible because it can spread around and it's the benign tumour you pray for. In neurosurgery that distinction is anything but obvious. Sometimes more important than the type of cells that form the tumour is its location. A benign tumour in a very important structure of the brain can do the most damage.

For example, right in the centre, in the midbrain, the 'clockwork' of the brain which controls stuff like wakefulness, blood-pressure and breathing, a benign tumour can cause immense difficulties. Partly as it grows and squeezes important nerve endings, but also when we come to try to remove it. Accessing and then cutting at something in such a delicate area is like walking a tightrope. The odds of injuring an important structure can be greater than the chances of removal.

The majority of tumours present by affecting the brain around them and causing a problem with the function. So we may see children who have developed a weakness in the limbs or poor core balance, or difficulties with eating or with vomiting after they eat.

Problems with their speech, their vision. Anything that you can think of that the brain controls can go wrong if there's enough pressure on the cells in charge. Seizures are common. Even something like epilepsy can be a result of a growth muscling in on the brain.

It gets worse.

While tumours that grow from outside can constrict the brain and do serious damage, they do tend to be more easily removable. Sometimes, when you've removed such a tumour, the brain will expand back to fill the space.

With those tumours the biggest question is the quality of the boundary between the tumour and the brain. If it's a very good one, as in 'this bit is brain, this bit is tumour' and they're just lying next to each other rather than entwined or incorporated within each other, then you can hope to achieve a fairly clean break. Other than the brain vessels coming in to feed the tumour, you can work carefully around the whole lump, cutting it up piece by piece.

In brains, and in children especially, those neat little packages are rare. The worst types are what we call 'intrinsic' – that is to say, they're within the brain itself. Not next to it or around it, but part of it. The issue then is how much brain tissue is within the tumour as opposed to how much tumour tissue is within the brain? On the edges of the tumour, how much is the interface between tumour and brain? How well delineated is it? How large is it? Can you make out brain from tumour with the naked eye?

There's one type of tumour known as DIPG – Diffuse Intrinsic Pontine Glioma – which grows within the middle or 'clockwork' part of the brain. It's insidious, completely embedded. Good cells grow networked with bad cells. They're impossible to separate. In those cases you just have to hope chemotherapy and radiation will treat the worst of it.

Imagine two hands together with interlocking, overlapping fingers. Where does one finger end and the other begin? Which one is a brain cell and which one is a tumour cell? All you see is tumour interwoven with brain. It gives you, as a surgeon, a decision to make. 'Do I cut off from the left knuckle? In which case I'm leaving those fingers of tumour behind. Or do I cut off at the right knuckle? In which case I'm taking all the tumour, but all those bits of brain as well.'

What we can't do is operate down to the cellular level. We can't go in and take individual cells out and leave alone those other cells in between. Chemotherapy can go some way towards a similar result, but the scalpel capable of the type of incisions necessary has yet to be invented. And neither, I suspect, has the surgeon.

The question is: what should this child's treatment comprise? While the decision will ultimately be mine and the family's, I like to take advice from my learned colleagues. Every week I sit down with the oncology, pathology and radiology departments and we work through the results for our upcoming and ongoing patients. With the right people it's a healthy and productive way to work. And, luckily, we have the right people.

I might have four or five 'hot' cases in the pipeline, each at various stages of treatment, and the oncologist will have a similar number. We present each case and use each other as sounding boards. At best we're trying to find the best possible treatment for each individual patient. At the very least we want to avoid the scenario where you've attempted a risky operation only for the radiologist to say, 'Why the hell did you operate? It was obviously a very chemo-sensitive tumour.'

Some situations are black and white. After a sample biopsy or a bigger removal, the pathologists will present the slides of what they've seen and say as categorically as they can, 'This is tumour X.' Then the oncologist will say, 'Okay, we now need to proceed with this type of treatment' or 'Let's do another scan because it looks like it's a GRT.' This means a Gross Total Resection – it's always so good to hear that we have removed the tumour completely. There's little to argue with following such assertions.

It's the cases where a biopsy has yet to be performed where opinions come more into play. Based on scans, the radiologists will give us the top two or three likelihoods. If their feeling is that a tumour is chemo-sensitive (one that will likely respond well to chemotherapy – drugs that we can give by mouth or injection) I take that on board, especially if the tumour is in a dangerous location. But if I can see that it's in a really easy-to-get-to-place with minimal risk to the patient, then sometimes I will advocate doing the operation. Why subject anyone to months of ravaging chemo when a 'short, sharp shock' style of treatment can get them on the mend in days?

It's all about consensus. About minimizing risk for the patient and providing the best care. Sometimes getting there can feel like a battle, but usually it arrives fairly organically. As it does with my latest case.

Scans show that the entire left side of Baby's brain is taken up by tumour. Malignant or not, I put her likely lifespan, if untreated, at no more than a fortnight. The oncologist agrees. As does the radiologist. And the pathologist.

The fact that the patient is so tiny, so frail – born a month premature – means she might not survive multiple invasions. Even if we had the time. But then again, she has about as much blood as in a small glass of wine in her whole body. We need to have a clear plan when to stop – and this is likely to be decided by blood loss. Again, it's a balance.

But it's decided. We're going in. And we're going do as much as we can in one hit.

* * ✦ * *

Of course, the parents ask me about the chances of success. They always do. I make it a personal point never to paint a rosier picture than we have. I don't pull punches. In this case I am not able to say that the success rate for this type of operation is high.

Later that night, I ask myself, 'Why do it?' We're looking at a patient who should, by rights, still be in the womb. What's the point of subjecting her to the nightmare of surgery if it's too risky? Surely she should have some chance at life. Her family should have some time with her, even if it's only days or weeks. Without a decent track record, it could be said that there would be no justification for putting babies or their families through that kind of agony.

Let's say I'm quietly confident we can help. But trust Dad to ask the one question I never answer. 'Can you cure her?' he says.

I shake my head. I won't ever use the word 'cure'. There are too many variables. So I say what I always say in these circumstances: 'We can certainly aim to *treat* her.'

The anaesthetist is ready. His heart-monitoring equipment has been bleeping monotonously for the last ten minutes. Two large screens stand between him and my scrub nurse. On one we have the scans displayed for reference. On the other is a live view from an ultrasound machine. Between my knowledge of anatomy and the image the camera will give, I'll have a kind of sat-nav to guide me through the brain.

First we have to get in. As Iron Maiden's greatest hits strike up, I shave the section of the baby's head that I need to access. Then I cut very carefully into the soft skull. At this stage, it's so soft that we can use a pair of scissors to open it up. Carefully, I lift off the pentagon of bone and see with my own eyes what the scans had already shown. Except it's not my own eyes.

You've probably seen the ridiculously exaggerated glasses that surgeons wear. If they look like little telescopes over each eye it's because that's what they are. They're called 'loupes' and come with immense magnification. Perfect for when a millimetre out of place can mean the difference between a patient walking or not.

The loupes sit low on the nose so I can see down at my work while being able to peep over the top at my colleagues and the information on the screens. I look up only occasionally, however, just to confirm I'm where the sat-nav thinks I am. Even then I don't move my head, just my eyes, for fear my hands will follow. It's enough.

The baby's brain is the size of my fist. It looks complete, rippled like a walnut. To a layman it's probably exactly everything you'd expect from a 'brain'. Except everyone in the room knows full well that around 50 per cent of what we're looking at should not be there.

We know, from our anatomical training, what those ripples should look like and where those ripples should be. Through the loupes I can make out where they become distorted. That doesn't always mean I'm looking at the tumour, just its impact. In this case it's both.

There are many ways to proceed depending on the work ahead. In this instance, I won't be using a scalpel. Not unless I need to. The patient is too delicate, the risks too high. Not so long ago we wouldn't have had alternative options. Luckily for us all, we do now.

The nurse hands me a thin cylinder attached to a cable, the tip about the size of the cartridge inside a Bic pen. It's an ultrasonic aspirator. It's actually two cylinders, one inside another. When held against a tumour, the inner cylinder vibrates at such a frequency as to disrupt and eventually dissolve the tissue. At the same time, a thin shaft of water from between the cylinders irrigates the area to form a micro-slush, and then a vacuum sucks up the liquidized result into the inner tube. It is without doubt the safest approach we have, easily the gentlest, and, at something like £40,000 per unit, among the most expensive.

And, I think, as I look at my 12-inch-long patient, *worth every penny for the lives it saves. And the quality of those lives.*

I begin the work. Before my magnified eyes the tumour begins to disintegrate. The first piece is bottled and sent immediately to pathology for analysis. Then it's back to hoovering up the rest. It's a satisfying process, like window-cleaning or demisting a car. You can see exactly where you've been and where you need to go.

I move from the outside edge inwards, occasionally flicking my eyes at the screen to check there aren't any vascular blood vessels or other crucial pathways hidden within the mess. Occasionally, I glance at the heart monitor. No change. Nothing out of the ordinary. Which is good.

For an hour I move the magic pen across the dubious mass. As I reach the border with the brain itself, I hear the theatre doors open. A registrar stands at my shoulder. The pathology results are in. 'It looks malignant,' she says.

'Thanks.' I keep working. But inside, I think *Bollocks*. I'm pretty sure I said it out loud as well. But we can't give up. Not yet.

I'm virtually done with the majority of the tumour. Now for the tricky part. Even with my super vision I can't make out where the lump ends and the brain begins. It's not the best analogy, but if you've ever sat with fussy eaters during a steak course, you'll often see them lopping off huge chunks …

'Why are you doing that?'

'I don't like fat.'

'That's not fat.'

'It is.'

'It isn't. Try it.'

Et cetera, et cetera …

With neurosurgery, you can't just 'try it' and then spit it out if you don't like it. The damage is done by then. Literally. But you can do other things. An ultrasound scanner is very good at picking up the subtle differences in tissue mass, which is key where there's a danger of blood vessels or major junctions. For example, at the spot where tumour and brain tissue meet.

The ultrasound sits directly on the brain. The pictures appear on the screen. One look up, one down and I shave off a couple of millimetres. Another look up, another down and a few more go. I can see a corridor of maybe an inch that should be safe for me to dissolve. When I get close to the join, I might need a microscope. Precision is all. I don't want to jeopardize Baby's function too much, if it is malignant.

I shave as close to the border as I dare. Further down the line, when Baby is out of the woods and strong enough, a course of chemo might be able treat anything I don't take today. The aim of today's operation is to remove the overwhelming pressure on the brain to the best of our abilities. We've done that.

It's all about playing the odds. And right now, as I declare our patient 'treated', those odds are in our favour. I won't know for sure how well surgery has gone until Baby wakes up, but I feel good about it. As I stand back to let my registrar begin the clear-up and the replacing of the skull piece, the dulcet tones of Rage Against the Machine scream in my ear. It's been a good day. Our work here has given this child, with an initial life expectancy of two weeks, an extended shot at life, an increased chance of being the baby daughter her parents dreamed of.

I'm satisfied we did all we could. More importantly, we didn't overreach. *I* didn't overreach. Aiming for the moon when you're still on the ground is very tempting, but it can have catastrophic results. As I know from personal experience …

CHAPTER SEVEN

EVERYTHING THAT MAKES US HUMAN

You can't trust me. At least that's what I tell my juniors. Same as I say I can't trust them. There is nothing in our line of work that doesn't benefit from a second pair of eyes or ears. If a registrar shows me scans, I'll double-check that they're the right way round. Then I'll get the registrar to do it. Maybe I'll even get my scrub nurse to look as well.

It's weird. At home I'm an untidy, slovenly mess. I'd sit around in my underpants and watch *The Simpsons* all day if I could. But at work I'm an anal freak. Mr Details-Upon-Details. I check, double-check, triple-check, quadruple-check everything. Then I say to whoever's in the room, 'You check it.' Even fundamental things like which side of the head the tumour is on get the Spanish Inquisition.

'Okay, scan says left side. Do you agree?'

'Yes,' says the scrub nurse.

'You?' I ask.

'Yes,' says the anaesthetist.

It's not that I think the guys in the MRI department can't do their job. I'm just not going to take anyone's word for anything if I can check it myself. In our line of work there's no going back. Patients don't have the luxury of us trying again. If I take something out, it stays out. So I give the same pep talk to everyone who works for me.

'Don't trust me just because I'm your boss. If you think that I'm about to do something wrong, something stupid, you shout. You stop me. I'm relying on you. What's more, so is the patient. Even teachers make mistakes. We're a team. We succeed as one and we fail as one.'

It's a heartfelt speech and a hard-earned one. When you become a consultant, it's not like you suddenly know everything. You've done six, eight or ten years. You've reached an arbitrary level of skill. But it doesn't stop there. The only way you grow is with experience. That means more operations, more patients, more learning – and, if you're human, more mistakes. Every surgeon, probably every health professional, has a debit and a credit column. The trick is to learn from everything. To try not to make the same mistake twice.

I'm not sure I've ever done anything a colleague would say was 'crazy wrong'. But I have made decisions that in hindsight could have been better. And one of those decisions I still think about to this day.

I said I never use the word 'cure' as a promise. But when we operate, we do need to try to remove as much of a tumour as we can. This is our job. Sure, if you're too aggressive you can needlessly cause injury to a patient – which they may endure for the rest of their lives. But if you're too timid, you will likely ensure that that life is needlessly short. So, knowing our limits is one of the most important things we learn. But it doesn't come easily. There is a general rule that the older the surgeon gets, the more cautious he or she may become. Perhaps it's natural as you collect a group of neurologically injured patients, sitting on your shoulders, as you progress through your career. But I was a young consultant at this time. Operating was the thing for which I'd trained for half my life.

If working on the potential child abuse cases in Toronto and back in Oxford had taught me anything, it was that you can never stop taking on other people's ideas. I devoured medical journals from all over the world, spent every spare moment scouring the Internet for new breakthroughs or suppositions. When I first became a consultant I read lots of articles about the American health system. Obviously it's predominantly insurance-based, but that aside their hospitals were reporting staggeringly high 'success' rates for brain tumours year on year. Our UK numbers, by comparison, were paltry.

I chatted it over with my mentor and senior consultant, Peter. 'Why do you think it is?'

'Well, obviously US hospitals are private, so they need to chase the dollar as much as any other business. Record-breaking success stories will get you funding, no doubt about it.'

'But why are they so successful? Why don't we have those numbers?'

He looked at me with a hint of disappointment. 'Because in this country we don't take risks with patients' lives for the sake of money.'

He was being controversial, but I felt maybe he was right. The NHS paid my wages like it had paid his for decades. There was no pressure on us to 'bill' big numbers at the end of each quarter. We had one job and one job only: to save lives. And yet, article after article kept saying the same thing: 'It's amazing, man. These guys are curing people. All hospitals should be doing that.' The stories really spoke to me.

I was young. I was ambitious. I was desperate to save the world. But the whole world didn't need saving. Not then. Not that day. Whereas the little guy with the parents in my waiting room did. I swore I was going to do everything in my power to help him not just survive today, but every day. I was going to try to *treat* him.

A cure would have been brilliant. I never told him that, I never promised his family that, but I explained to them that it was always a possibility.

'It's going to be okay,' I said. 'I've got this.' And I really thought I had.

Famous last words.

．　．　◆　．　．

I could just write about the cases where I've taken all the tumour out, the patient was absolutely fine and everyone lauded me as the great surgeon of our times. But those moments fade away, because however good your last case is you'll always then get another one which goes wrong and that keeps you very grounded.

A ten-year-old boy who today is still one of my patients came in with a very short history of problems with balance, coordination and headaches. He had a scan locally and it showed a brain tumour at the back of the head, in the cerebellum. He was pretty unwell – struggling, actually – so he got sent straight across to us overnight. He was here in the morning when I arrived. Mum was with him. She couldn't have been much older than twenty-five or twenty-six. Young and absolutely terrified could have described them both.

I explained what was going on, told them why they were here and said, 'The tumour is only going to do more damage. We need to go in and take it out.'

Mum was horrified at the idea of her son's head being cut open. The boy picked up on her reaction and started crying. I managed to calm them down, but stopped just short of saying, 'If you don't want to have the operation you don't have to.' Because, frankly, I didn't think either of them were in a fit state to make that choice.

What I did say was, 'Take some time to process it. It's a massive deal, I get that. You'll experience some pain and maybe some weakness and balance problems after the operation, as I've explained. And you'll take a while to recover. But the alternative is that we do nothing and you'll lose the ability to control your arms, your legs and eventually you will get sicker and sicker.'

And you die. Obviously, I didn't add that bit, but Mum got the message. Reluctantly, she understood what had to be done.

'Tell me honestly, though,' she said, away from the bed. 'What are the odds?'

I don't really like to encourage false optimism, but from what I'd seen on the scans this was as close to a home run as could be.

'I'd say the risk of anything going seriously wrong is low, perhaps five or ten per cent,' I replied.

Any gambler would snatch off both arms for those kind of odds. But I'm dealing with parents. What do they care about the ninety fit and healthy kids running around if their child is in the 'unlucky ten'?

'Okay,' Mum said, very apprehensively. 'Do it.'

The tumour sat plum in the fourth ventricle, the area that controls so many vital structures and functions such as heart rate, blood pressure control, breathing, even consciousness. All the wiring that comes from the brain down to the arms, the legs, everywhere, goes via this tiny little area. The good news was that it looked pretty accessible. As, in fact, it was.

The surgery took most of the day, but I managed to get the tumour out with no complications or problems at all. Sometimes they're like that. If you get a clear run at them you can grab the whole lot, fourth ventricle or not. Led Zeppelin get some of the credit. They supplied the soundtrack. But I felt good, too. In surgical terms we'd done a clean extraction. It couldn't have gone better.

Bouncy as we all were after a successful op – hard not to be with 'Whole Lotta Love' blaring in the background – I wasn't getting too carried away. I always need to see the patient awake and responsive before I light the metaphorical cigar. With this chap, though, I thought it was only a matter of time. But it turned out that it was a long old time.

When we tried to bring the patient round, the doctor from the Paediatric Intensive Care Unit (PICU) realized there was an issue with his conscious level. He wasn't breathing for himself and wasn't waking up at all. When I got to his bed I was surprised to see him still asleep. The soft whirring of the ventilator attached to his throat was all I could hear.

'Has he woken up at all?' I asked the ward doctor.

'No.'

'Is he triggering?' I wanted to know if he was trying to breathe through the ventilator.

'Nope. He's not responding.'

'Okay. Give it another couple of hours, then do me a favour and get him scanned.'

'Will do.'

They ordered a scan. We waited as each slice of the sixty-four cross-sections of the imaging came up on the screen. The most important ones were the last ones, of course. But it looked great – a textbook result. On the images, that is. But I wasn't treating the images.

He wouldn't wake up, so we left him on the ventilator. Without the little tube sticking out of his mouth, he wouldn't have been able to breathe at all. Obviously, the mouth is used for more than breathing. In order to feed him, the doctors had inserted a nasogastric tube directly into the stomach.

He was completely unconscious and remained so, without any anaesthetic medicines, for days, then weeks. He had a tracheostomy – a hole was cut into his neck, and into his airway, to allow a long-term connection to a ventilator. He had a PEG tube – a feeding tube that punctures the stomach and comes out through the abdominal wall, like a mini-Alien. This allows liquid feed to go straight into the stomach, and then the face is completely clear of any tubes. A face that does nothing.

What was the cause of this disaster? The scans looked great – no stroke, no bleed, not even any obvious large remnant of tumour.

If there was any left, it was just a tiny bit. But there was no other explanation. Even if I didn't know the reason for the present circumstances, it must have been me.

In my desire to treat the tumour, I must have caused, unnoticed, some damage to a microscopic but crucial vessel. To the naked eye it would have looked like a tiny vessel feeding the tumour. But it must have been one that went inside the tumour and out the other side and actually fed the brain, not the bad stuff. That's why I was going so slowly, so carefully, taking off such tiny fragments at a time. But I had to be sure. I went over every piece of video footage from the operation and couldn't find the crucial moment. I spoke to my assistant, the scrub nurse, the anaesthetist. They had no idea when it had happened. There had been no change in patient status throughout.

Peter could see I was torturing myself. His attitude was that I'd set out to treat a patient with a brain tumour and I'd achieved it. There will always be risks, potentially fatal ones, when you open another living being's skull. Brains were not built to be toyed with. There's a reason they come packaged in a solid bone case.

'These things happen, Jay,' he said. 'The feeling of guilt will take time go away, but you did nothing wrong. You do your best. You use every tool at your disposal and every lesson you've learned. And you help where you can.'

It was a difficult conversation to have, but there was another even more painful. Telling the boy's parents what had happened and what I thought had gone wrong was very challenging. But I also needed to explain things to my patient. It took weeks before he even started to show any inkling of waking up. As soon as he was conscious, I stood at his bedside and broke the news as gently and coherently as I could. It was heartbreaking watching his earnest little face stare up at me, unable to speak, unable even to nod or shout or scream.

As always in these cases, the family turned out to be stronger in some ways than me. They pointed out that at least their son didn't have cancer anymore. I'd treated him for a tumour that would have killed him eventually, for which they were grateful.

It was true. He didn't have a tumour. He didn't have cancer. But he didn't have any quality of life either. Everything that makes us human had been stripped away.

He underwent intensive rehabilitation. Eventually, he was transferred to a long-term, specialist rehab hospital. There aren't enough of these, and he had to wait months for a space. From there, more months of difficult relearning of the most basic functions awaited him. He remained with a tracheostomy and PEG for several years.

◆

That little boy is now fifteen years old. Over time some significant functions returned. He still breathes through a tube, but he can speak and has mobility in his arms and torso. I see him every year for check-ups and each time there's a miniscule improvement.

The one thing that has altered, however, is his attitude. From the moment he was first able to communicate before leaving us after the operation, he blamed me, the hospital, his family – everyone around him for where he'd ended up. He was so angry and hated himself as much as us. We had to spend a lot of time helping a young man, just a child really, learn a whole new way of life. He couldn't be expected to understand why we needed to do this operation. All he knew was that he had some headaches and came out of surgery basically paralysed ... or 'wrecked' as he described it later on.

Over time, though, as he has got older, he has gradually learned to accept his situation – he's still angry, of course, but he's different. Now, when I see him and tell him what he knows anyway, 'it's a tough, long haul', 'you can't give up, keep working at it' and other rather useless sounding platitudes, I get more of a teenage grunt, a shrug, and he's away in his wheelchair. Occasionally, he'll give me the finger as he leaves my clinic. But at least I have been able to give him the good news. There has been no tumour recurrence – the bit I left behind must have given up the ghost and died off. It sometimes can do that. And it's been long enough to now count him, officially, as 'cured'. When I told him that, he said drily, 'Yay, so I get to live even longer like this. In a wheelchair, not even being able to go to the toilet by myself. Thanks so much, Jay.' Not much I can say back to that really.

He certainly changed me at the same time as I changed him, though not necessarily in terms of my surgical approach to cases because there was no fault in procedure. The crucial blood vessel that had been damaged could have been snagged at any point, not just when I was going for the brainstem. I guarantee that it's happened to every neurosurgeon on the planet. If it hasn't, then they aren't doing enough cases. Or aren't treating them properly. You can't see things that don't want to be seen.

It's more about changing my attitude. I've grown to see the value of a quality life rather than just a long one. That little boy who never walked again would be dead by now, 100 per cent, without that intervention. As it stands, he'll probably see out his parents, as all kids should. But here's the question: would you prefer five years of a quality – 'normal' – life, knowing there's a clock counting down somewhere, or would you rather have decades, albeit severely impaired?

It's not a distinction they teach you at med school. Doctors are meant to heal. We fix. We patch up. We keep alive. I can't remember the lecture where they discussed not doing anything and just watching the patient die. Maybe they teach it now, but not then.

Of the many, many cases I've worked on, a fairly high proportion have fallen into this area. I've found myself having the discussion with parents and, in some cases if they're old enough, with the children. How much does quality of life mean to you?

Interestingly, a lot of parents can't cope with the idea of putting a finite limit on their child's life. They want me to go all-out, guns blazing, to rid their child of the killer disease. They just want their son or daughter to survive at any cost.

Others take the more pragmatic approach. Sometimes it's just the fact of being in hospital for tests and appointments that swings the balance. One parent told me, 'Doctor Jay, we really don't want our daughter's life to consist of coming in and out of hospital every five minutes. We want her to have a normal life for as long as we're allowed.'

They're not alone. Perhaps surprisingly it's the patients who tend to agree with them most. Children are very good at knowing what they want. And most of them don't want to have to keep seeing my ugly mug when they could be playing with friends, going to school, or arguing with their siblings like anyone else.

· · ◆ · ·

Complications happen. Over the course of thousands of neurosurgical procedures that's inevitable. It's human nature that those are the ones you tend to remember. They're the images that flash into your mind as you're about to doze off by the swimming pool on your summer holiday. They never really leave.

It's not that you don't remember the good-news stories. They just don't stay with you. I don't lie awake at night remembering all the lives I've transformed, all the little boys and girls wandering around who wouldn't be if it weren't for me and my team. I mean, who apart from the patients and their families cares?

Imagine: 'Read all about it: Highly Trained, Highly Skilled Neurosurgeon With Loads Of Experience Saves Patient!' It's not exactly front-page news. It's basically a man doing his job and not cocking up. Don't we all strive to do that?

I know how easily the success stories are forgotten because I didn't just work on one patient the day I overreached. On theatre days it's standard practice to fit in two or three cases, usually one 'big' one, and couple of smaller, less time-consuming procedures. Something like reducing the build-up of fluid inside the brain can be over in eight or nine minutes. The album version of Lynyrd Skynyrd's 'Free Bird' on my theatre sound system lasts longer than that. On that fateful week where an errant blood vessel changed the course of a boy's life, I also worked on another little person. This time with better results. Certainly with better luck.

· · ◆ · ·

It's another boy and he's four years old. He has a tumour in the middle of his cerebrum, the big main part of his brain, next to the fluid space known as the ventricles. I'm hoping this one will be over quick enough so I can squeeze one more case in. Because we don't have an operating list everyday with our paediatric anaesthetist, we need to be efficient with our time, while being safe.

How long the procedure takes, though, isn't up to me. We don't even know what we're dealing with. Scans show where the tumour is, but not what it is. I've decided that I won't go full invasive immediately. 'Let me drop a scope in, see what we're dealing with, and try to get a bit for the pathologists first. If it needs to come out, I'll get it out. If it can stay where it is, we'll do that.'

It may seem strange to suggest that, but again it's all about risk and benefit. It might be something that looks odd on the scans, but has been there for ages. The child presented with a seizure, caused by the lesion (the term we use when we aren't sure what we are dealing with) irritating the brain next to it. That can be treated with anti-epilepsy medicines. It's difficult to know for sure – some things can look different in real-life patients from the pictures in textbooks.

We have taken samples of blood already to see if we can detect any hormones. Some tumours secrete hormones that are basically diagnostic, meaning no biopsy is needed. The bloods were normal, but something still looked funny about this lump.

I only have to shave the smallest area of hair then drill a hole no more than about a centimetre in diameter. It just needs to be wide enough to take the endoscope. It's another bit of kit that Peter never had growing up in neurosurgery. At least not anything this compact and reliable. The endoscope is basically a fibre-optic camera in a stiff probe. It has a channel within that lets me pass instruments down it, and so it can work in the middle of the brain without opening up the whole head.

I feed the scope through the hole, my eyes never leaving the large screen overhead. At my suggestion, the young trainee next to me calls out everything he sees. 'Passing through the skull, dura, into the brain, into the ventricle.'

I rotate the camera. 'What do you think?' I ask. 'Do we need to take the lid off and go in guns blazing?'

He studies the picture. 'The tumour is pushing on the side wall,' he says.

'Good. What do you suggest?'

'Biopsy? See if it's malignant?'

'And what else?'

He pauses. 'I don't know.'

'Well, is the patient in immediate danger if the tumour is benign and we leave it?'

'No, boss, it looks like it's been growing without too many problems for some time. It is possible that it could go ages before we see serious implications. But we need to know what it is, to be able to plan the next steps. So I wouldn't just pull out. I would defo do a biopsy.'

I pass a needle through the endoscope and enter directly into the tumour. It takes a sample of the lump, then junior rushes it up to pathology. The phone call comes twenty minutes later. We turn down Talking Heads, so I can hear.

'Good news or the bad news?'

'Bad,' I say. 'Always bad first.'

'It's malignant.'

'Okay, and the good?'

'It looks like a germinoma.'

This is exactly what I was hoping for – a type of tumour that can be treated without surgery. And one with a really good prognosis. I look at my assistant with a 'What do you think?' kind of face. He gives a thumbs-up. Correct answer.

I guess he's possibly disappointed not to assist on some major skull-cutting and drilling. I would have been at his age. But even with the American dream of 'cure, cure, cure' still buzzing in my head, I'm happy to wrap up and pass my patient over to oncology. There have been enough Normandy Landings here for one week.

CHAPTER EIGHT

WIGGLE YOUR BIG TOE

L ike a lot of parents, I have an office pin board and desk that are filled with artwork from my children. Every so often I'll look at a drawing and try to remember what it was meant to be. It changes depending on my mood.

Not all the pictures are from my own kids. I've got sketches from dozens of children, all patients, some of them going back a decade. More than a few seem to be caricatures of me. Is there anything as critical as a child-artist's eye? It's a nice way to remember the wonderful people that pass through these doors. Not all of them come back for annual check-ups. Not all of them are still alive today, but in every single case we gave it our best shot. I get a lot of cards from parents that say 'Thank you for trying'. I'm not sure I could write that message in their circumstances, but it means a lot.

Every year, around the second week of December, I receive a card from one particular man. He wishes me a 'Merry Christmas' and thanks me for fighting so hard for his son. I've received fourteen of them so far. He never forgets. For a parent, the experience of the neurosurgery department never goes away.

Children like to mess around. It's what they do. They're attention seekers and it's the parents' job to sometimes ignore them.

If your four-year-old started stumbling around, your first thought would not be that maybe he has a major spinal disease. You're more likely to laugh or tell him to stop mucking around and get up to the table for dinner. Maybe the next day he complains of a sore tummy and you say, 'Well, when was the last time you did a poo? Let's go to the toilet.' When he wets his trousers later, despite being dry for over a year, you're just relieved he's urinating because getting a wee out of him has been nigh on impossible over the last twenty-four hours.

When you realize he hasn't jumped on your bed at 6 a.m. you might actually be happy. You might cuddle up to your partner and enjoy the privacy for once. But when you creep over to check on him at 7 or 8 o'clock, you don't find the sleeping bunny you expected. You see him wide awake, on the floor, distress in his eyes.

You run over and scoop him up. 'What's wrong, baby? Why are you on the floor?'

'It's my legs, Daddy. They won't work.'

The young boy had been taken into A&E at Northampton with a retrospective four-day history of worsening walking, sore tummy and urinary incontinence. He also couldn't take any weight on his legs at all. They quickly realized it was a spinal problem – a job for us at the John Radcliffe Hospital. The on-call trainee at the time, Tim, received the message and took down the details.

'I'll get the boss,' he said. 'You get the boy over here ASAP.'

I used to operate two days a week. This was not one of those days, so there was nothing in my diary that could not be shifted. Tim ran me through the story.

'What's your best guess?' I asked. I already knew what *I* thought it was. The way trainees become consultants is by calling the decisions themselves.

'Either a tumour or some bleed into the spinal column,' he said. 'Anything else?'

'Possibly an acute MS attack?' Sometimes, 'medical' conditions like multiple sclerosis can look like a tumour.

'Yeah, it's possible but unlikely. One of the first two will almost certainly be the culprit.'

The MRI results came through and confirmed a problem with the spinal column. The boy had developed an arachnoid cyst. It's benign in and of itself, but it can cause disruption to the flow of signals in the spinal cord. Over a period of probably months, perhaps longer, it had been growing but with negligible detrimental effect. It was only over the previous few days that it had reached the tipping point, grown too large for the available space and started compressing the spinal cord. It needed to be drained. Pronto.

Neurosurgery has three theatres in its name. Sometimes – often, in fact – we need one more. At that moment they were all in use. All doing great work. I didn't want to bump anyone's operation later in the day, but this was an emergency. I made the call.

'Theatre eight: how long till you're finished?'

'Just started – three hours.'

Theatre 11: 'Four hours minimum.'

Theatre 12: 'About sixty minutes.'

'Perfect,' I said to the last theatre. 'Once you're done, I have a cord compression I need to do ASAP. Can I have your list?'

There are two types of surgical colleagues. Some whinge and complain, and do everything they can to avoid giving up their space to someone else's emergency. Others say, 'Yep, if it needs to be done, it needs to be done.' Fortunately, this consultant was the latter sort.

We did the WHO surgical checklist. 'We are getting prepped for spinal cord decompression. Thirty minutes till he should be here, people.' The anaesthetic consultant led the WHO and drove things forward in theatre. With a scrub team already on site that was one less thing to worry about. Now I could focus on the actual patient.

The boy's cyst was located between the shoulder blades, which explained why his arms were still functioning. As for everything below, he was paralysed or soon to be. Not just the legs, but the bowels and the bladder and everything else south of the problem was a target for the block.

· · ◆ · ·

The ambulance arrived within an hour of the call to Tim. The parents were in turmoil. Self-flagellating at missing or dismissing every sign. They were begging everyone, 'Please, help our son. We'll do anything, sign anything. Please help him!' It's natural. I'd deal with them shortly. First, the priority was giving their child the once-over. Northampton had inserted a catheter into the boy's bladder because he could not pee. It was up to us now – physically and mentally.

· · ◆ · ·

In a non-emergency – for example, when it's somebody coming with a long-term condition that will be the same tomorrow as it is today – the protocol is that one of my juniors would be first contact for the family. They perform the introductory hellos, run through our projected care plan and become the patient's person of contact. It's not me skipping on tasks – I'm not treating patients the way my father's heart specialist treated him – but my job is more than saving lives. It's about training the next generation of specialists. The trainees need to learn, so they're just laying the groundwork before I arrive. It's my version of 'see one, do one, teach one'.

The registrar examines the patient, takes a full history from them and their carers, and comes to me with a summary of what they've found, plus a formula of what action they're recommending.

Normally, I will already have seen the scans so that I can make sure they – we – are on the right track. I want to see whether my trainees are on the same page as me. Real world experience counts for more than any exams. That said, it's as much to make sure that I haven't made a mistake as it is checking the trainees.

It's the same process I underwent and I think I turned out okay, the odd blip aside. But another reason for sending your troops into the field is much more positive. They're young, they're bright, they're hungry – so they may well come up with a better idea than anything their forty-something boss has got. Sometimes you have to say, 'You know what? That isn't what I was going to do, but it sounds great. Let's do that instead.'

Whether we go with my diagnosis or not, usually I like to get the trainee to come in and do the operation with us, so they've got that ongoing link with the patient. They tend to remember much more if they have continued involvement.

When things are in motion in a rapid way, concessions need to be made. I'll go down with the trainee and we'll see the parents and child together, and then normally one of us will peel off to the operating theatre to tell everyone there what we're planning to do, what kit we'll need – what playlist I'm in the mood for. The other person, meanwhile, would be getting the consent forms signed by the child or the parents.

Because of this boy's situation, 'training day' goes out the window. There's no time for standard techniques. This was a case of everyone seeing the family together and then everybody going off and making their contribution to processing the next part of the next stage. Time wasted now could mean reduced limb function later.

◆

I'm standing over the boy, checking his notes, making small talk. He is conscious and scared. Dad is right next to me. The second I turn away from his son he mouths to me, 'Please. Be honest: is it cancer?'

'I don't think so, no.'

'Oh, thank God.' He and his wife hug. They cry. I can feel the palpable relief, of course.

I really want to let them enjoy the moment. But that would be unfair. 'It's not cancer,' I say, 'but it is serious.'

'What do you mean?'

I explain what has been found. The large fluid-filled sac is compressing the spinal cord and has almost completely stopped the signals passing up and down. The longer it goes on, the more likely it will be permanent. 'I mean, your son might not recover his lower body functions – legs, bowel, bladder, sexual function – all of it.'

Dad's face tightens. 'Please, Doctor Jay, not in front of my son. I don't want him to hear this.'

I acquiesce and step away from the bed for a second. But not because I agree with him. Dad is close to breaking. He just wants me to save his precious boy's life. I want to ensure it's a life with as little pain as possible, which also includes mental discomfort.

I explain my diagnosis to the parents and give a rough outline of the surgery we're planning to perform. I don't pull any punches.

'We're going to try to save your child's legs and bladder function as much as we can. It will either be successful or not. Function may only come back a little bit. It's impossible to say at this moment. The only thing I can guarantee is that if we don't operate, if we don't take a chance right now, it will only get worse.'

The parents are strangely happy. Everything's fine. They just want *someone* to do *something*. It's the only way they will be able to live with themselves. But telling them what I plan to do is just part of my job.

'Now,' I say, 'I need to tell your son.'

'Absolutely not,' Dad replies. 'He's too young for this.'

It's the usual story. Normally, I'm a little more reasonable. *Normally, I have more time.* 'Wouldn't you want to know what was happening to you?' I ask.

'Of course. But he's a child.'

'Yes, he's a very *scared* child. And it's my job to help him in any way I can. And right now, that means explaining to him exactly what we're going to do. I can't envisage what horrors he's experiencing right now. Imagine being four years old and your legs and bum have stopped working. Imagine not being told that someone is going to inject you with sleep drugs, then waking up with a sore back and a tube hanging out of your spine. Personally, I'd be terrified.'

'I don't know,' Mum says.

'I'm sorry, time is of the essence here. I respect your opinion, but you must respect mine,' I reason. 'Trust me, I've been doing this a long while. You will cause more damage in the long run by keeping secrets. More importantly, he is my patient, not you. I'm not going to lie to him.'

It's harsh, but we're against the clock. Children have voracious imaginations. Imagine what hellish scenario he could construct after waking up with no information? It doesn't sit right with me. There's only so much four-year-olds can take in, but I want to share the basics. They are reluctant but agree to me talking to him.

'Your legs and tummy are controlled from your back. And that is what isn't working properly. We're going to give you lots of medicines that will make you sleep and then we'll have a look around inside your back to see if we can fix your legs and tummy – we need to get them back to work, don't we? When you wake up you'll have a little bit of pain, but that will go away in a day or two. You might have a little tube coming out of your back. It will feel weird but it won't hurt. And we'll take it out as soon as possible.'

With the help of Benny the bear – the ward operation toy we use to explain to children what will happen to them – I show him what we are planning to do.

Best-case scenario: the lad wakes up all discombobulated, head spinning, wondering where he is. The pain receptors will start to kick in, he'll be uncomfortable, he'll be aware of something in his back, but he'll think, *Oh hang on, Dr Jay told me this was going to happen. He said I'd feel sore but that I'd get better in a day or two. So that's okay.* Even at four years old, knowledge is power.

. . ◆ . .

The surgical scrub team are waiting when I arrive. Two anaesthetists, an anaesthetic assistant, my trainee, one scrub nurse, two other nurses and, as often is the case, a handful of students. Students aside, everyone knows what we're planning to do, the equipment is ready, they've just completed another life-saving op. This is bread and butter for them. If anything goes wrong it won't be their fault. I'd bet my life on it.

I'm in theatre ten minutes before my patient arrives. The anaesthetic room is next door. Completely separate. I can hear his trolley being wheeled in there. The team are getting him comfortable and administering the knockout juice. As a rule of thumb, ambulance staff and relatives and other hospital personnel are admitted into the anaesthetic room, but that's where their access ends. Theatre is a clean environment. It's my environment. Things that go wrong in here, even if caused by other people, ultimately have to be explained by me to the patient and their family, so I am jealously protective of it.

The patient is wheeled through and put on the operating table. We position him with great care, making sure we look to protect any pressure points to keep the skin safe. Then we do the flight checks. Tim hands me the scans.

'Confirming the right way round,' I say, waiting for it to be verified. 'And confirming child's name.'

It sometimes seems like a waste of time checking the identity of the patient against his charts, but accidents have happened. Not to me, thank goodness, but the wrong leg has been amputated because scans were pinned up back to front, and occasionally the wrong patient has ended up under the knife because of a mix-up over similar surnames.

It happens. But less so if you run the relevant checks.

We go through the cleaning techniques, applying antiseptic and antibiotics. Finally, we're ready to start. I set up the sound system – the music kicks in. Getting into my operating brain thoughts, I scrub up.

The task is to drain the errant fluid pressing on the patient's spinal cord. We're all clued up and primed to go. The boy is lying on his tummy. I cut a vertical incision into the middle of his back, slicing through the skin down through the muscle on either side of his tiny spine. Once I reach bone it's a matter of clearing space. My scrub nurse then hands me the drill required to open the back of his spine.

The aim is to drill in such a way as to allow me to lift off a sizable length of spine, like a link bracelet. The incisions I'm making are approximately 10 cm long. It may not sound much, but it is seriously invasive in a four-year-old's back. A few millimetres too far left or right and I could damage the boy's spinal joints. Too deep a penetration and it could be worse.

By cutting down the side of the spine I can ensure the ligaments hold everything in shape. It's intricate stuff, but so satisfying when it works – a bit like peeling an orange in one go.

The spinal cord sits inside the bony vertebral column. It's completely surrounded in fluid and fat to protect against impact. That means as you move, your spinal cord doesn't get bashed against the bones of your spine. Much like the way the brain is cushioned inside the skull. If you have a sudden increase of back-up fluid in between the spinal cord and the bones of the spine – caused by a cyst – you can imagine what a snug fit it would create. You'd have this fluid sac growing bigger and bigger and bigger, and eventually it would tip over the edges into what we call 'decompensation'. Suddenly, the spinal cord doesn't have enough blood supply because it's being compressed so much and it starts to prevent bodily function.

It's like travelling on the Tokyo subway network. Just when

you think that there's no way you can get another person into that carriage, a guy with white gloves comes along and shoves several other bodies inside. There's no room. Everyone inside is squashed. Breathing is difficult. Dignity goes out of the window. But still they cram more people on.

The actual cyst I'm searching for is probably half the thickness of my little finger. As I lift off the link bracelet of the boy's spine, it exposes the fibrous bag – or dura – surrounding the spinal cord. Aided by the microscope magnifying the tiny operating field, we open the dural sac, and use tacking sutures to hold it open. It's a win. I can see the cyst as plain as day, very prominent, packed with clear fluid. The aim now is to open up the cyst and drain the fluid out, but also to try to 'fenestrate' – where we cut as many holes as we can in the wall of this cyst – so that it can't refill.

With one puncture we could have drained the sac, sewn the boy up and waited for him to regain some semblance of function a few days later. In doing so, however, we'd be inviting future complications. Whatever is causing the cyst and the fluid build-up within would continue to do so. Within six months, the boy would be back reporting similar symptoms.

So that is why it's not enough to make one hole. I have to make several – half a dozen if I can. The body has this annoying habit of healing any scars – usually a good thing, but in this case an inconvenience of life-changing proportions. Make two holes and the body might heal one within six months and the other in a year. Make six and you'd have to be seriously unlucky for them all to heal.

Voodoo needlework done, I stitch up the dura, then lower the link bracelet of the spine down and secure it into place. It has to slot in perfectly to maintain the integrity of the spine's biomechanics. If it's misplaced, a growing boy could end up with curves in his spine or other problems.

It takes an hour to rebuild the jigsaw and close. Everything is finally connected back to where it was before. Confident we've done as much as could be expected, I call an end to the surgery. The scrub team can then prepare for whichever operation they were meant to be doing for the last couple of hours. I need to speak to my patient's parents, then wait. And wait.

· · ✦ · ·

I have never guaranteed a surgical outcome. By the same token, I've rarely intimated results that were anything other than likely. I'm Mr Middle of the Road. I believe that patients should be as informed as I am. No hyperbole, just plain probability. I'd warned this little boy that we may be able to reverse his condition, but it was by no means guaranteed. I'd told his mum and his dad the same thing.

The whole procedure took about four hours. The patient was declared safe and moved to a ward. We'd started late afternoon and it was the middle of the evening by the time we were done. On a non-surgery day, as today originally was, I should have been home in time for family supper. If I rushed, I could possibly still catch the dying embers of the meal. But as tasty as the boss's cooking is, I couldn't leave without updating the parents.

'We've done what we set out to do,' I said.

'Have you fixed him?'

Ah, the most common question. 'We've disrupted the sac, but the spinal cord is a very intricate part of the body. We should have stopped the damage progressing, but I don't know if we will see an actual improvement.'

Slowly, the boy stirred. I tried to get him to move his legs, but there was nothing. *Still early days*, I thought. He was so tired after the ordeal of the day that he nodded straight back off to sleep. That's enough for one day. I said goodbye to my team and the parents, and hit the road.

The following morning I did my ward rounds as usual. There were eleven cases within our purview, each of them as important as the next. Everyone was as I expected them to be, even the ones in the ICU. Two I was able to sign off for discharge. Another pair I prepared for surgery later in the day. But the person I was secretly most anxious to reach filled me with nothing but disappointment.

I said 'Good morning' to Mum and Dad and then my patient. It's always important to include them in any discussion. I asked how the night had been, then opened the question up to the nurses. 'Anything you need to report?' I asked.

The nurse in charge replied that there was nothing of import. 'Temperature standard, heart rate normal, sleeping pattern regular. No leakage from the wound.'

The boy was awake, smiling in between bursts of discomfort, which always gives hope to the coldest of hearts. But when I asked, 'Can you move your feet for me?' his reply was 'No'.

'Are you sure? Are you sure you can't wiggle your big toe?'

He stared down at his feet and concentrated. Nothing happened.

I touched them gently, but he couldn't feel them either. He was exactly the same as his preoperative state.

'It's okay,' I said, as much to his parents as to him. 'It can take some time.'

The following day produced the same response. Dad was beginning to go crazy. He wanted a result.

'As I said, the surgery went as well as we anticipated. How it manifests itself is less clear. But it's early days.'

'Early days? How long are we expected to wait?'

'As long as it takes.'

Every day I walked the wards and every day it was the same story. 'Can you wiggle your toes?'

'No.'

'Are you sure? None of them? Can you wiggle your big toe?' It's stupid, but every time I ask someone to do that, I remember it being said in Quentin Tarantino's *Kill Bill: Volume 1* film. Except in that case it's the patient, played by Uma Thurman, ordering herself to do it.

Anyway, back at John Radcliffe, he couldn't. 'That's okay. There's always tomorrow.'

As each day passed by, Mum became more resigned, more sanguine. Dad, by contrast, was increasingly wound up. He wanted answers, he wanted results. 'When will he be able to run? When will he cycle? When will he be able to take up boxing?' At least that is what came out of his mouth. What he really sought, however, was absolution. He was haunted by the idea that he was responsible for his son's condition. 'Why didn't I listen to him when he said his tummy hurt? Why didn't I notice when his walking changed? Maybe if I'd woken him up an hour earlier, then we could have picked it up an hour earlier and you might have saved something.'

It was as painful watching him torturing himself as it was registering zero improvement in my patient. Nothing was Dad's fault. It's human nature to say to a child who's complaining about anything to 'run it off' or 'go to the toilet' or 'get an early night'. They're all quick fixes that tend to work more often than they don't.

'Listen, there was absolutely nothing you did wrong. How on earth could you have known this was going on? You need to forgive yourself and spend your energy on him. It's early days,' I reassured him. 'We have to be patient.'

Rehabilitation is as much about your state of mind as it is about your state of body. You've got to really work at it and want to work at it and put the effort in. Whether you're four years old or forty, it's all too easy just to lie there and go, 'Ah, it's never going to happen.' And you'd be right. We know that the psychological state of a patient has a direct relationship to the recovery they can enjoy. We tell patients that they 'need to stimulate the nerves back into action'. But what four-year-old can do that with a father chuntering 'It hasn't worked, it hasn't worked'? I wasn't just working on my tiny patient. I had to treat Dad as well.

Four days turned into five, turned into six, turned into ten. I was so concerned at that point that I ordered another set of scans. What if a blood clot had occurred on the operation site since I'd been in? That could explain everything. But there was no sign of this. It all seemed fine.

On day eleven I made the same pass through the building. Mum and Dad barely looked up when my team and I swanned in. *Eau de guilt* filled the room. My solidarity with my patient's parents was being tested. I would have given anything to have them feel less guilty.

'Good morning,' I said, just as I'd done on the previous eleven days. 'Do you have any news for me?'

'No,' my young patient replied. 'Sorry.'

'That's all right, completely okay. But as I'm here, could you just try to wiggle your big toe for me? If you can't you can't, that's okay.'

I'm not sure I was even paying that much attention. It was mainly the reaction of the boy himself that shook me into life. He was giggling, laughing, pointing.

And why? His big toe was wiggling. Just like Uma Thurman's in 2003. In fact, all of his toes were moving. The extremities of both feet were alive. It was crazy. The most heroic scene that ward had experienced for ages.

Yes, you could say it's a relatively miniscule part of the body. But the toes are also the furthest from the brain. If the signal is forcing its way down to them, through whatever blockage there had been, then there is a very good chance it is reaching out to the various points in between. In this instance, legs and possibly bowel and bladder.

But that was getting ahead of ourselves. Right now we had a small win on our hands. I was choking with happiness. My trainee and other staff were besides themselves. Mum was gobsmacked. Dad looked like he just wanted to cuddle someone. Of course, his enthusiasm didn't stop there. 'Come on, let's get you up and walking!'

'Please,' I said, 'you have to give him time. Some people in his condition regain control of their ankles and that's it. That's where it stops. You can't force him without making him feel bad.'

He looked so contrite. 'Yes, yes, of course, you're totally right.'

As it turns out, and not for the first time, I was totally wrong. It was like turning on a tap. When I swung by for the next morning's meeting, I was thrilled to see a young boy sitting upright and looking downright bored. He had significant function in his legs. In twenty-four hours he'd gone from wiggling his big toe to flexing his ankle, bending his knee and arching his hips. Remarkable progress even for us old pros.

He was discharged after about three weeks. I was confident by then that full motor performance had returned to his legs and elsewhere. And how did I know? Because on his last day at John Radcliffe he walked, unaided, out of the door. Some days are full of sunshine. We save such memories to balance out against the rainy ones.

Just because you're out of my ward, it doesn't mean you're off my radar. Every six to twelve months, most patients call back in for check-ups so I can monitor progress and see how the physio is going and whether the rehabilitation is on track. Sometimes everything is so perfect that we say goodbye after a year, sometimes three years. Sometimes it's ongoing forever.

Four years after this lad hobbled back to Northampton, he visited me for the final time. He could barely remember a time when he couldn't walk as well as everyone else. If it weren't for my notes I'm not sure I'd have believed it either. Happily, I have no need to see him ever again. But in the meantime, there are the Christmas cards.

CHAPTER NINE

THE TESCO TEST

There are very few times when the music goes off. Often, I have differing tastes to my colleagues and team (in fact, swap 'often' to 'always', and 'differing' to 'totally opposite'). If I am doing something that really takes my concentration, then I need to hear music. Generally, colleagues know that and they leave the sound system alone. Sometimes, if we are doing a less demanding procedure, the team will sneakily change it to a different playlist. I can usually manage to cope with something more socially acceptable – I think I am getting better at this now that my kids force me to listen to the streaming version of the Sunday afternoon Top 40 (how I fondly remember those days – finger ready on the 'tape record' button).

There's only one scenario where the soundtrack gets unplugged and I don't complain. In fact, it's because *I've* shut it down, which is never, *ever* a good sign.

◆

A child's head isn't solid skull. When you're born, you've got various plates that make up a skull and there are growth lines between them. Often, you'll see the middle part of a baby's head – the diamond-shaped area known as the fontanelle – pulsate up and down because there isn't actually bone there. It's part of the membrane in which the bone grows. It's a bit like ice forming in water. The plates of bone are like ice and they grow towards each other over time.

The bone itself is fairly firm. But the joining bits, the membranes, are quite soft. They need to be for two reasons. Without the plates of the bone being able to ride over each other, the baby's head could never make a vaginal delivery. It would be too big. The second thing is that those junctions between the different plates are where more bone can be laid down and the skull can grow. The growth during the first two years is beyond rapid. By the time you're two, your head size is about 80 per cent of an adult's.

If you think of the changes that a child goes through in those first two years, the demands of a massively expanding brain, it's no wonder the skull needs to grow so quickly. Whereas a baby giraffe, for example, comes out of its mum pretty much fully wired because it can walk and feed independently, human babies are useless. But not for long. They go from being completely helpless squishy things, to angry, sometimes-capable-of-shouting-back-and-throwing-stuff squishy things in no time at all. They crawl, they eat, they communicate, they toddle, they develop fine motor skills – they become tiny people exceptionally quickly. Nought to sixty in a matter of months. No wonder David Attenborough calls them the most impressive creature in the wider animal kingdom. A lot of remarkable brain development occurs in a brief time period – and the plates have to keep up.

But what if they don't? What if those junctions between the different plates fuse too early? It's called craniosynostosis and it happens, sometimes while the baby is still developing within the womb. If it does, it can create a small but firm head that is still able to be delivered normally. More often the plates will fuse after birth. But whenever it occurs, it's often bad news. If the whole skull fuses as one, then there is total restriction of head growth. If just a section of the junctions start to harden then, as the brain demands space to develop and expand, other parts of the skull will grow in compensation. So instead of pushing on the left, for example, which it now can't do because there's fusion of the suture, the brain pushes double strength on the right, resulting in a distinct distortion in the shape of the head.

Of course, many babies have 'funny-shaped' heads when they pop out, especially if forceps or other tools have been used in the birth. Parents may not initially spot an issue, being so excited about their little new addition. A midwife sometimes will. If the problem doesn't kick in until later, then it's the parents who are most likely to notice it first. Luckily, with the power of the Internet, at the slightest concern they can hit Google, do a bit of research, print off a sheaf of papers and quickly run things past their health visitor or GP. Sadly, the medical profession tends to switch off when patients say they've seen something online. I can see why: a simple headache can seem like a brain tumour on certain sites. But parents do tend to know. More than a few have arrived at my clinic saying, 'Thank you for taking me seriously. Everyone else said I was a paranoid, crazy parent.' Easy for me, though, isn't it – the diagnosis has already been made.

Whether the problem is picked up pre-birth or ten months afterwards, there's often no real point doing anything about it until around the twelve-month mark. Though it's true that for every day you delay treatment there's the chance of pressure building inside the restrictive prison that is the skull, operate too early and you'll only have to go back in and repeat the process further down the line. It's not a universally accepted time frame, if I'm honest. Compared to a lot of units around the world we do tend to do ours relatively late. But our procedure is much more extensive and definitive, I would say.

If physical signs aren't recognized, then behavioural flags can be. If there is a problem with pressure inside the head, then babies can become irritable, not want to lie down, not sleep properly. Sometimes their feeding goes off. If it's particularly serious, and goes from symptomatic to developmental problems, then they can start to miss their milestones. Maybe they're not sitting up at the age they're expected to. Or they're not reaching out when they should do. They might not be growing at a reasonable rate. Perhaps they have problems with vision. Particularly in genetic or inherited cases they may get double vision and not develop the ability to have 3D stereoscopic vision.

Regardless of the tells or the family history, it always boils down to the same thing: a skull meshing too early and often squeezing the brain. And that's when we're called in.

Our next patient was six weeks old, referred to us from another hospital with the note: 'This baby clearly has craniosynostosis.' The plan was to get her into clinic in the next few weeks, observe, check and make a plan. That was all agreed when the other hospital first called us.

They phoned back after a couple of days. 'Actually, it's more than craniosynostosis. She's started vomiting a lot. Can you see her earlier? We'll transfer her across to you. We think she has Crouzon's syndrome.'

Crouzon's is a genetic condition in which there's a change to a specific receptor on the cells of the skull that affects the way the bone is laid down. It means you get rapid fusion of the skull sutures as well as changes in the brain anatomy, opening the door for hydrocephalus – a build-up of fluid in the middle of the brain. So not only might you have a small skull, which can raise the pressure inside itself, but the hydrocephalus can also increase the contents of the skull through the build-up of water, thereby raising the pressure even further.

We had a look at her. Clinically, it appeared that she did have Crouzon's syndrome, plus problems with pressure inside her head. When you've got fusion of the sutures, the brain still needs somewhere to go. If all of the sutures start to fuse, in actual fact, the weak spot starts to become the centre of the plates of the skull rather than in the joints. Even though the bone is hard, and the brain is soft, the brain starts to wear away the bone as it pushes slowly out, just like water eroding rock.

The head takes on a very classical shape as this wee mite demonstrated. It can become quite small, wide on the sides and tall at the front. The head is described as a clover-leaf skull because that is the shape it grows to look like. Obviously, these changes take time, much longer than six weeks. Clearly the transition had begun *in utero*, building up for months possibly. But, just as clearly, we knew it wasn't a case that could wait twelve or eighteen months.

As well as the build-up of pressure, I was worried the baby was susceptible to Chiari malformation, and not a mild version of it. This is where the bottom part of the brain (which should remain in the skull) pushes into the top part of the spinal canal, causing compression of the important brainstem structures and contributing to blocking the fluid pathways, hence the hydrocephalus.

There were problems with the growth of her face and therefore with the airways through the nasal spaces. We could expect breathing problems resulting in a tracheostomy, especially if her face doesn't develop properly. Babies are already quite snuffly by nature. It doesn't take much to restrict their already small airways.

It's not always my decision which operations get bumped. All I can say for sure is that this baby became top priority as soon as she arrived.

We've done the ward rounds, which featured me, another consultant, two plastic surgeons, nurses, registrars and trainees. We've done the WHO briefing. I know everyone I'll be working with and they understand what we expect. And as hard as it was to tell them, so do the parents.

We're not about to embark on a quick fix. There's no easy remedy for what Baby has. We can make a difference, that much I can be sure of, but how much? Plus, it won't be easy and it won't be quick. The operation we're about to attempt will be the first of many. The various physical and functional problems caused by the syndrome are still going to be there when Baby wakes up. They will be for the rest of her life.

Today is just the first of multiple operations, all designed to allow the brain to grow and to give the skull and the face functionality. A secondary hoped-for outcome is to improve things from an aesthetic perspective. Basically, we want the child to pass what we call the 'Tesco test'. I don't know who coined it, but it means that when she's old enough, I want her to be able to walk around a supermarket and hold her head up.

The first operation in a series carries more weight than the rest. We need to find a way to give space to the brain but without screwing up the operations further down the line. Everything needs to be meticulously planned, as it's not enough to map out just what we're going to do today. We've had to sketch out the whole of the next ten years of her life, which is why we work so closely with craniofacial plastic surgeons. In this case it's my friend and colleague, David Johnson.

The Chiari malformation and the compression of the back of the brain needs urgent attention. The bone has worn away so much that it gives the appearance of fingers, mere slithers of carapace. In between is a more supple substance, but it's not just dura. Some of it is actual brain.

Every heartbeat makes the brain pulsate a little, pushing against the inside of the skull. Despite the obvious difference in consistency between bone and brain, the bone is slowly worn away by the brain. The surface of the brain is rippled. The outer parts of each ripple – the mountains, if you like – called the gyri, wear away the adjacent bone first. In what we call the sulci – the dips or the valleys – there is less wear, so fingers of bone are left. Eventually, the gyri overlap and integrate these fingers of bone into the brain structure. The skull can look like a pepperpot – which is what we call the condition.

The stakes couldn't be higher. We have to get those fingers of bone out without damaging the brain underneath and around. It's complicated by the number of abnormal veins protruding from the back of the head. One misstep with the scalpel or dissectors and they become serious issues. At best, the veins might bleed. If they are major enough, they may cause a backup of blood in the brain and then a stroke. At worst, they'll start to suck in air.

Anyone with a GCSE in biology knows that the heart is designed to hold blood, not air. Damaging one of these veins would be like sending air directly towards it on an expressway. One minute you're dissecting the bits of bone, the next you have an air embolus on your hands – and within seconds, a potentially dead patient.

Think of deep-sea divers. If they surface too quickly they get an overload of nitrogen bubbles in their bloodstream, which can lead to lung problems and bring on a stroke and even be fatal. A baby on an operating table can experience exactly the same thing without getting its toes wet. Air in the bloodstream is like putting soap liquid into water. It creates bubbles that get pumped to the lungs, which then start to block off the blood flow in that direction, giving you a massive problem with oxygen delivery. I'd like to say it's all just theory. Things you learn and hopefully avoid. But right from the get-go it's all I can think about.

We make the incision into the scalp and the next step is to peel back the layer of skin to give me access to the skull. The scans are set to larger than life on my screen. I peep over my loupes to check once again for any veins in the cutting area. There are none flagged. Even so, I am constantly watching for any changes or bleeding as David makes the cut.

It goes to plan. We fold back the skin and begin phase two. I'm using very fine dissectors and an instrument similar to a microscopic spatula with which to lift the brain, then trying to nibble a bit of bone away with a small pair of pliers. It's really slow, meticulous work. A drill would fly through in no time, but the risks of error are too great. This has to be done by hand, bit by bit by bit.

With every clean strike I inwardly breathe a sigh of relief. But if anything it only piles on the pressure. Each next movement seems to carry more danger, the greater likelihood of an accident.

We've been going nearly two hours when suddenly the anaesthetist says, 'This isn't good.' Sumit Das is one of the best craniofacial anaesthetists around. Terrible taste in music, but he knows his stuff where it really counts. If he is worried, we all should be.

We pause. Look at him. Listen to his machines. The heart monitor sounds erratic. Something has gone wrong.

'Change in oxygen levels,' Sumit calls out. 'Blood pressure dropping.'

'What's going on?' I ask, already knowing the answer.

We start dripping then pouring water over the head, to avoid any more air being sucked in. 'Air embolus.' Even as he confirms my suspicions, he's attaching a syringe to Baby's drip.

'Adrenaline,' he announces, and starts to feed it into the patient, trying to provoke a response.

Nothing. In fact, worse than nothing. There's a high-pitched continuous bleep. Exactly as you hear on every medical programme. The kind of bleep that means only one thing: flatlining.

'Bloody hell!' he says. 'She's arresting.'

Several things happen at once. The first is that the music gets shut down. I don't have to ask. I certainly don't complain. I couldn't hear it anyway. The most obvious reason for the heart stopping is that we've caught a vein. David folds back the scalp as I continue flooding the area to keep the puddles of water where we want them. It's fast, frenetic, reactionary. But nothing compared to what the anaesthetist is doing.

His job, at its most basic level, is to monitor the patient's heart rate and keep it comfortable. He doesn't expect to be doing it manually. He's got his hands underneath the little sheet covering Baby. His fingers are locked around the spine, leaving his thumbs free at the front for tiny but firm chest compressions. He starts to press and count. Press and count. Too hard and he'll snap the rib cage and possibly damage the lungs or heart. Too soft and he won't trigger a pulse.

Everyone knows what they're doing. We discussed this likelihood during our pre-op gathering. Even so, dealing with it is something else. We're all matter of fact. Calmness personified, at least on the outside. There's only one goal: bring Baby back to life.

I've done as much as I can at my end. David and I watch as Sumit, his head barely a foot from mine, works away. Thirty seconds come and go. I'm beginning to feel the pressure.

'Right,' says Sumit, after a while longer, 'let's stop and see where we are.' He leaves his hands in place, but stops compressions. There is an eerie silence as we all look at the screen. I hear something. It's a beep. A small, faint beep. Followed by another. And another.

I look at the anaesthetist. The sweat is pouring off him. He checks his machines. He takes his hands off Baby. He looks at me. And he says, 'Panic over. Let's try not to do that again, shall we?'

I've said that a good scrub nurse runs the theatre. The surgeons oversee the actual operation, but only up to a point. The anaesthetist is the one looking out for the patient's overall well-being. I'm the one who decides what we do, but the anaesthetist is the one who decides what we *don't* do.

After a flatline situation there's always a bit of analysis, a bit of reparation. He'll try to carry out various treatments to get the heart rate and blood pressure into workable positions. If he has any doubts at all, he can call the operation off. In this instance, I think more inexperienced anaesthetists would have done. They'd have panicked.

Our guy doesn't. He knows us. He's aware that we'd discussed causing an air embolus as a possible outcome and he was ready. The worst had happened and we dealt with it as a team. Once satisfied that Baby was stable again, he saw no reason why the team couldn't continue. Which we do – without further problems.

I say 'we' because in this case the other consultant in the room, David Johnson, is about to take over. My task is to assist with taking the bone off the back of the head, these islands of bone, all the way down to the junction between the skull and the spine. We call this 'pepperpotting of the skull' – because that is what the skull looks like – with multiple holes in it. It went right the way around the head, and by releasing the restrictions at the back, we can take the pressure off the brain.

If it's my job to remove the errant bone and protect the brain, it falls to my expert consultant colleagues from the plastic surgery department, like David, to run most of the show. They make the skin incision and peel back the skin from the skull, plan the layout of the new skull, and put the bone back so as to create a bigger skull for the brain, and then close up. Except we don't put it back in this case. I've already thrown away all the 'fingers' of bone. We are left with a space the size of my palm, which on a six-week-old baby is quite substantial, but David just stretches the scalp back over the affected area, essentially leaving no bone over the back of her brain. We needed to leave room for further growth. Our next operation, when it happened, would be as much as a year away thanks to this procedure.

It's quite hard to imagine a large boneless part of your skull. I mean, how do you lie down? Surely you'd notice the soft bit at the back of your head? Fortunately, babies never seem to realize. I suppose everything else in the skull is so soft that they don't recognize when the skull ends and just skin continues. You hold your breath when you see them lie back, but they don't flinch. It's amazing, really.

Operations like this involve such close work with the plastic surgeon. I've known many over the years. They're all incredibly gifted and driven to help. They're not just in the business of cosmetic improvement, although of course they do facelifts, tummy tucks and boob jobs. They're here to give patients a shot at a normal life. To help them to pass the Tesco test.

We would go on to do seven operations jointly over five years on this child. Each one was designed to bring us closer to that goal. Each one essential.

It's not only the skull under the hair we have to worry about. Children with this combination of conditions also have very small faces. Their facial bones are extremely restricted in growth. Without intervention, Baby's eye sockets – or 'orbits' – would naturally remain small as she aged. That was the case until she reached two years old. Then we did an operation on the front of her head.

To the strains of Black Sabbath, I remove Baby's forehead and the upper parts of the orbits around the eyes clean off, as though I were lifting a pair of spectacles. David then refashions them into larger 'glasses', and essentially we reshape and reposition this bone further forward on the skull. I find the whole process fascinating. I'm as much a student as anyone. It's the plastic surgeon who maps out my cuts and is in charge of piecing the shapes back together into a new-look skull. I'm just a highly paid carpenter.

The result looks a bit extreme until the rest of the face catches up. It also leaves gaps between bone pieces, which we pad with crumbs of sawn-off shards, then re-cover with the skin. The joy of the human body, though, is that the gaps will be filled by fully formed bone soon enough. It certainly makes our job easier.

With the children who are suffering from some genetic causes – so called syndromic craniosynostosis – it's less about worrying over any gaps; we're actually praying it doesn't fill too fast. The whole reason for their particular condition is that it lays down bone too rapidly.

On Baby, we worked on the top part of the face first. In theory you could deal with everything at once, but it's wasted time. Until children have their final 'adult' face, you'll be redoing it again and again. It's only around eight or nine, maybe ten, that you get a real sense of what they're growing up to look like. Only then do you have something concrete to work with, and the final facial growth will sometimes only happen in the early twenties.

The whole process is hard for parents. I'm talking about from six to eight operations, but these aren't back to back. They're over a period of years. The parents and the patient have to live in the interim with a fairly different look for the child. And it's not as if each operation is an obvious step forward. When we moved the whole 'spectacle' section of Baby's head forwards, it didn't look exactly right. But we weren't doing it to improve her for that day or even that year. We were putting the infrastructure in place for her long-term maturity. She was literally going to grow into her face.

The advantage that parents have is knowledge. Being forewarned is forearmed, as they say. Some mums and dads, for example, are at work one day and they get a call to say their child has been hit by a car and is in intensive care. As regards the consequences, there's sometimes no warning, no getting your head around it or preparing yourself. It's a complete rug-pull.

On the other hand, when a child is born with a 'medical' condition affecting their skull structure, the issue is flagged early on and the fixing process is slow and methodical, so there's plenty of time to adjust.

When we first sat down with Baby's parents, it was a case of saying, 'Your child's skull isn't developing normally. We're going to take steps to adjust, but it's merely the start of a long, long walk. Our priority today is to protect her brain function. Then we'll work on her appearance – she might need or want further surgery to help her find her ideal place, if that's what we all agree is needed. It shouldn't be that a child should have to undergo surgery to conform to what the rest of the world thinks. But then again, it's easy to moralize if you aren't the kid getting bullied, the teenager left out of meet-ups, the adult feeling too shy to talk to someone special at the office party. It's not going to happen overnight. But we will get there.'

At least that was the gist of it, but it took many hours to have that conversation. It starts with us saying hello in clinic, or on the ward. We go through everything so far, a full history and examination is done. Then we discuss the condition for a while. Later, after a break, our nurse specialist comes back. She goes through everything again – sometimes people like to ask her questions they feel might be too mundane to put to us. The ward nurses, all fantastic people with a wealth of experience, also help to discuss the recovery from operations. Play specialists may help with anxiety for the older kids, some of whom know exactly what's going to happen to them and are distinctly unimpressed.

In some cases, where the patient has just one single growth line that's fused early, we're able to cut some of the skull out, reshape it, put it back together and hey presto – it's done. We meet at clinic once a year, but usually that's all that's required. We might stay in touch for fifteen years and never do anything other than chat. You just never know.

More serious 'plain neurosurgery' cases will stay in my orbit for eighteen years. The follow-up is as important in some ways as the cutting and shaving. It doesn't matter what level of treatment you get. You're my patient until you stop being a child and beyond. From birth to voting age. And even after then, I guarantee I'll be sticking my beak in and checking your files when my colleagues in the adult wing take on your case. However, craniofacial patients don't get moved on – we keep them. Since we really are experts in their conditions, there is no benefit in transferring their care to someone who does less of this work.

One of the things I say to parents is, 'We're not looking for perfection. Not everyone out there can look like Angelina Jolie. God knows, I certainly don't look like Brad! What we want is for them not to stand out.' And that might sound like a low target, but think about all the people you see on a day-to-day basis. Look at your fellow travellers on your daily commute. How many stand out as beautiful or attractive or something special? Very few, I suspect. The rest of us just sort of jog along, nothing special, no one's looking twice. We're not going to win Sexiest Man Alive – and we're not going to turn milk sour by looking at it either.

My goal is simple: I want my patient to be able to decide what he or she wants to do in their life. And to do it without feeling restricted because of the way they look and the way they function. I want them to be comfortable at school, at social functions as teenagers, at work. Maybe they'd like to go out to bars and clubs – chat people up, find a partner, get married. Maybe they don't. The point is, I want the decision to be what they *want*, not what they feel they are able to do because of how they look. I want them to be happy people. It's what we all wish for our children. And if I want it for my own offspring, then I want it for all my kids.

Obviously for the more severely affected patients, brain function can be an issue that becomes more apparent over time. Parents start to notice the difference between their child and others, not only physically but developmentally. Perhaps they are slower to move forward in school, they need one-to-one attention, sometimes even special schooling. That's much more difficult for families to cope with. Baby's parents were typical. They weren't worried that she was slower to learn than her peers. They were looking ahead. 'What's going to happen to her when we're gone?' They never stop caring. Never stop putting Baby first.

One of the things I most admire about the parents of the children in my care is their optimism. Baby's parents weren't just brilliantly attentive, always ready to fight her corner and look after her every special need. They asked me one day, 'Do you think we should risk having another child?'

I would never, ever give advice about whether two people should have another baby or not. It's not my place. But I will and do and did point out the risks. However, since we have one of the world's most famous craniofacial geneticists on the payroll at John Radcliffe, I'm able to say, 'Don't take my word for it …' Such experts can give a percentage chance of a second or third child suffering the same condition as Baby.

Some families won't take any risks. They stick, as it were. Others twist. Ask to be dealt another card. Usually it's because they just want to bring children into the world. One family, however, told me they needed a healthy child to look after its brother when they were gone. It seems harsh on the younger, as yet unborn, sibling. But I can understand the logic, I think. I've seen enough of families to know nothing is guaranteed with siblings. Bloodlines alone don't always impel people to take care of their own family. Until it happens, you'll never know.

It doesn't exist in neurosurgery, but I've certainly read about parents of children with metabolic conditions, who need stem cells or organ transplants for example, who will genuinely have another child for the sole purpose of creating a potential donor. It doesn't happen often, but enough to register in the news. It's a very interesting ethical position to be in. I guess some people may think it's terrible, but unless you're in that position, you have no idea how you'd react. Maybe these parents were always planning on having another child. Who can be sure?

If I've learned anything from a lifetime in medicine and two decades in neurosurgery, it's that people are completely unpredictable with regard to their reactions. Some of the most sensible people who cross my path make the most irrational decisions. Others, often really young, seemingly quite immature parents, stun me by their totally logical approach that embraces all that is thrown at them.

I don't know if I could survive the unbelievable turmoil that some of them go through. Lots of my families do not come through it as a cohesive group. The separation and divorce rate among my parents is very high. Occasionally, couples are just holding onto a relationship, and then on receiving some difficult news about their child, it's less a case of a straw breaking the camel's back and more of someone landing a whole bunch of cement bags on the camel. So, no surprise there. But other families arrive rock hard and get destroyed by the emotional stress. It's either guilt or anger at the other partner for something they did or didn't do. I've actually heard some mothers say to their husbands, 'If I hadn't had this baby with you he wouldn't have had this condition.' Harsh, in every possible way. But health problems for children trump everything, even common sense.

Years later, I saw 'Baby', now a young lady, in clinic. 'Well,' I said. 'How did it go?'

She stared at her feet. Mum looked about to burst with pride.

'Well, she was in the shop for half an hour. I was beginning to get worried. But out she came with a bag full of sweets and ice lollies and the biggest smile. No one looked, no one stared.'

I smiled. Baby had passed the Tesco test.

CHAPTER TEN

SHE'S CONING

If you think about high-speed traffic that drives towards a town on a motorway, as it gets closer to the town the roads get smaller and smaller and the speed gets slower and slower. Then, as you drive out of the town, the road gets bigger again and the speed of the vehicles picks up and then you hit the motorway and you're driving at the limit. That's how the blood travels to and from the brain. As it gets into those intricate nooks and crannies to supply the oxygen, it's like a side road, the little street where people pootle along at 20 miles per hour. When it leaves, it's doing the equivalent of 70 mph, flat out.

That's the theory and, for most people for the majority of the time, that's the reality. But what if overnight someone builds a big bypass right into the centre of the town so you don't have to go down those tiny, windy roads? Nice in theory, but your car is going to hurtle in doing 70 mph and hit the centre without slowing down.

It's the same story if the blood to the brain doesn't have a chance to slow down from the full pressure of being pushed from the heart before it gets funnelled through the small, dainty blood vessels designed for lighter traffic. The good news is that road-traffic changes could never happen so quickly. With the brain, though, it's a very real possibility.

An arteriovenous malformation (AVM) occurs when there is a change to the way that vessels develop in the body. This results in high-pressure blood flowing straight into small arteries. This in turn results in unsustainable pressure on the vessels, which can cause rupture. It doesn't happen often in such a dramatic way – headaches or seizures are common ways of leading to a diagnosis. On this occasion, however, it was a full collapse.

My registrar took the call from one of our satellite A&E departments and ran straight to my office, collecting Tim, my senior trainee, en route.

'We've got a four-year-old girl coming in, unconscious. Scans are reported to show bleeding in the middle of the brain.'

'Have we got the scans?'

'On their way. But there's another thing. One pupil dilating.'

'Crap.'

A single pupil enlarging is a really bad neurological sign. When we shine a light into your pupil it's to monitor brain function inside. If you see both pupils appearing large and then shrinking with the light, that's a positive – it's what it is meant to do. It is the equivalent of squinting your eyes when looking at the sun – to stop too much light getting in. But if they become sluggishly reactive to light, that's a bad sign. If they don't react and stay large in size, it can mean that the patient is at risk of death.

'Okay, we're not going to have much time here. Are you up for this, Tim?' I asked. It was the old 'see one, do one, teach one' ethos at work. The only way for trainees to learn the hard stuff is to do the hard stuff. Obviously, I'd be standing right at his shoulder.

Tim nodded. 'Yup.'

'Great. Then you get a team ready. I'm going for a pee.' If there's the potential for a long operation, make sure the old preparation adage is remembered: empty bladder, empty colon, full stomach. I just needed one bit sorted.

According to dispatch, the ambulance was less than twenty minutes out. The scans arrived and confirmed a massive haemorrhage. A blood clot had formed in the middle of her brain and blocked off the path for the brain fluid. I could make out the abnormal collection of blood vessels from the AVM. It looked severe but we didn't need to deal with it straight away – it was the raised pressure that was the risk. If we didn't get a drainage tube in to deal with the build-up, the little girl was looking at devastating brain damage – if she lived. With every minute waiting for the ambulance, the prospects of survival were looking less and less positive.

What would normally happen in this scenario – scary as it was – is this. The anaesthetists would have everything ready on their side. The moment the ambulance gurney comes flying through the double doors, they'd be primed to go. The girl would be lifted onto their bed and the paramedics would fade back, their role done. All checks completed, the anaesthetists would wheel the patient the 30 feet into the operating theatre where we'd get her onto the table, position her carefully and begin prepping. We'd put a safety drape over her head to ensure it's all nice and clean and that we're not touching the skin, then we'd drape the whole body and give her antibiotics. Next, we look at the scans. Do they match the last ones we saw? Is it the correct identity? The whole first thirty minutes is all about providing as safe, aseptic and clean an environment as you can – and ensuring it's the right patient. There's always extra worry when people are coming in from outside, as all the usual preparations and inspections that would have been carried out on the wards haven't been done.

Checks completed, we would begin with the full anaesthesia, the precise incisions, the peeling back of the skin and run a bipolar electrocautery charge to minimize scarring afterwards. So many things we would do if we had the time. But from the second the ambulance guys burst through our double doors, I realized that was precisely what we didn't have.

· · ◆ · ·

'Pretty sure she's coning,' one of the paramedics calls out.

Damn. 'Coning' is shorthand for the clot piling up so much pressure that the heart rate centre at the base of the brain is being squashed. As it gets compressed, the heart rate drops and drops and drops. It's only a matter of time before irreversible dysfunctions arise.

'Heart rate?' I ask.

'Thirty-five and dropping.' He checks again. 'Thirty-four.'

Heart rate dropping so precipitously means one thing: imminent death. We're against the clock.

'Okay, guys, change of plan. We haven't got time to eff about here,' I say to the anaesthetist. 'The second you tell me, we're going in.' I am seriously worried that the time and movement involved in getting her onto the operating table will be enough to finish this poor girl off.

'We don't have time for theatre,' I tell my registrar. 'Get everyone here.'

Suddenly, it's a circus. The trolley crashes through the doors of the anaesthetic room. The gasmen are trying to keep the girl stabilized. Tim and I are splashing antisepsis on our hands, and all over the girl's head. I'm just in my blues. The room isn't sterile, there are people who've literally run in off the street. But none of that will matter to this little girl if we don't get going.

The anaesthetist has never worked so quickly. It doesn't matter that the girl is in a coma. We have no idea if her pain receptors are awake. She still has to be kept under like anyone else. And that takes time. The calculations are done on weight, but the standard amount of morphine and opiate sometimes isn't right for everyone. He needs to rely on his years of skill to estimate how much she needs and ensure that there is enough, plus probably a bit more.

Tim is alongside me. 'Sorry, mate,' I say. 'I have to jump in here.' 'Totally,' he says.

We both know the score. In any normal situation, Tim would have performed the op with me observing and no one would have batted an eyelid. He could even handle what was needed here, but in an emergency, with risk of death a near-certainty, the head honcho is expected to step in. If something does go horribly wrong – if the child doesn't make it – then the parents take some comfort from knowing that the 'best' people were on the job. And that means the senior person there. Me.

The truth is, my trainee is as capable of doing what needs to be done as I am. But my career is up and running. My reputation is made. The last thing I want to do is to expose him to the wrath of grieving parents, or lawyers, for something that is not his fault.

The ambulance guys step away. They're not getting their trolley back any time soon. This is happening now.

The anaesthetic room isn't built for visitors. It's tiny. It's already got the anaesthetist, his assisting ODP (operating department practitioner), plus me, Tim and now my scrub nurse squeezing in from the other side, dragging in the most essential theatre equipment. But it doesn't matter where we are. I'm still looking at a human head. This is all the room I need.

The second I get the all-clear, I make a stab incision at the top of her head, on the right side and to the front. It's the less dominant side and it doesn't tend to influence speech, so it's far less likely to suffer lasting damage from an invasion. There's no point in saving a child's life if she has no life worth living afterwards.

I make an emergency drill hole through the skull. Then I can see the dura – the fibrous bag enclosing the brain. I cut a hole and pass a ventricular drain – a silicone rubber tube – into the brain. I have to get to the fluid spaces which have been pushed over by the clot. We don't have scans in front of us. I'm doing it by memory. Muff this up and the game is over.

'We're in,' I say, as I feel the telltale change in resistance as the tube goes in from the school blancmange of the brain into the water of the ventricle.

The second the first drop of liquid hits the end of the tube, I glance at the monitors. Worst-case scenario: no change and we're too late. Best-case scenario: instant reaction. Which is exactly what we get.

'Heart rate rising,' the anaesthetist confirms, 'and the blood pressure is dropping.'

His voice sounds matter of fact, but his face is as elated as mine. Then the smiles fade and the mental exhaustion kicks in. Adrenaline is a wonderful thing, but when it crashes it really crashes. It's a more subdued room as we finish up. By the time we're done, the emergency is averted but the little girl is still unconscious.

'Now,' I say, 'it's time to meet the parents.'

Half an hour from start to finish. Transferring her to theatre would have taken another twenty minutes minimum, which is vital extra time that I guarantee the little girl did not have. Our mission was to save her life. The crash-bang-wallop-style procedure appeared to have achieved that. When she became stronger we would have to look at the ongoing cause, the AVM, and sort out the tangle of blood vessels. But that was for another day. First, she needed to live.

She was taken to the Intensive Care Unit (ICU). Often the registrar or trainee will do the handover, but as operating surgeon I wanted to complete the journey myself. After all, that was where the parents would be able to see her.

The ICU is its own department, just as mine is. It's not somewhere I would expect to waltz into and start barking orders, even though some surgeons still think they could. I handed over my patient and my notes and we went through everything we'd done, all that had taken place and, crucially, everything I would ideally like to happen next. For example, blood pressure kept at certain levels, heart rate regulated, coma induced – there are many options. They can only ever be requests, however, because patients don't always behave as you'd like – even those under anaesthetic or in induced comas – so the doctors and nurses on hand will make the calls they need to make. A lung problem or something else might reveal itself and they'll have to change tack. All the different specialities have to work as a team. At the end of the day, everyone has the same goal in mind.

In this instance, I suggested an ideal blood pressure, plus the obvious monitoring of brain pressure. Despite the coma, we had her under full sedation to help recovery. I suggested trying to rouse her within the next twelve to twenty-four hours, whenever they felt conditions were best. That was, I said, if she made it through the night.

Having explained it matter-of-factly to my colleagues, I then had to find different words to help the little girl's mum and dad understand what had happened and, more importantly, what still might.

Mum had been at home when the girl had slumped. She travelled in the ambulance and Dad had joined them at A&E. From that moment, I don't think they'd stopped crying or asking, 'Why?' It was almost a relief when they asked me the same question, because the answer is one of simple medical fact. I explained how the AVM had delivered the blood right into the sensitive blood vessels in the middle of the brain and how this had caused them to rupture and flood the area. I explained how we'd drained out the excess fluid and were monitoring their child.

But I also had to be honest about her current situation: 'Your daughter is not out of the woods yet. The next few hours are crucial.'

'What are you saying?'

Obviously, the girl had arrived in a very precarious state, which they knew. If I were to be totally frank with them, I'd have said that her chances of survival were 50/50 at best. Things could go very wrong very fast because the vascular malformation was still in there.

Not only could she succumb to the pressure she's already endured, but she could re-bleed again. With the brain already sick, then it could be a real disaster.

But those aren't the terms that parents want to hear. They deserve better chosen, more human words. 'I'm saying I'm really, really worried about her. If you've got other members of family who would want to be here, I recommend you call them tonight.'

'Are you telling us she is going to die?'

'I can't predict what might happen. She might die. She is very ill. We've done all we can for the moment. Now it's up to her.'

· · ◆ · ·

It takes a while to switch off after a traumatic evening, but the forty-minute drive home helps. That rubbish-filled car is my decompression chamber. By the time I step through the front door I'm almost ready to face being a husband and dad again. Even so, the first thing my wife asks me is never, 'How was your day?' She knows to skip that question until the first ten minutes is out of the way, just in case …

Obviously, between dinner and TV and playing with the kids and hanging out with my wife, the tiny flashes of memory of the day's emergency replay from time to time. I've no doubt that we did all we could. That's not the issue. So, I find myself thinking about how she is going to fare. I can't possibly know. It makes no sense fretting. It's not like I can do anything now. Of course, if something should develop, I'd want to be the first person my team called in an emergency. But fortunately no call came.

· · ◆ · ·

Driving into Oxford the following morning, I started to plot my day. Of all the patients I needed to see, there was one who I was most interested in at that moment. No news could equal bad news. I wouldn't know until I arrived.

I quickly got up to speed in the handover that occurs every morning. The real information would only come when I saw her myself. Ward rounds are the thing of myths in movies. In reality, they can be quite chaotic, as juniors try to catch up with results, listen to what we are saying to patients and think about potential grilling questions. Consultants couldn't do without these rounds because we need to be personally involved in the day-to-day progress of our patients, and face-to-face meetings are the best way.

I already knew before I approached her bed that our four-year-old patient had yet to wake up. But, as I said to the anxious parents and their gathered clan, it was great news that she had survived the night. The plan from here on in was to give her another twelve hours, then accelerate the waking process.

The great news, in my opinion, was that both pupils were now responding to light. The brain imbalance had settled. It wasn't quite the rise of Lazarus that the family was expecting, but I did my best to reassure them.

'We have to take the small victories,' I said. 'Just getting through the night was a massive achievement.'

I returned twice more throughout the day. I wanted to see with my own eyes what, if anything, was happening. The fact that I couldn't do anything more didn't impact on the family's gratitude that I was there. It's just human nature. In fact, nurses were checking on her and altering medication every half an hour. I, however, was the one they wanted to see. It's a lot of pressure, but something I don't mind doing. The family are my patients, too.

I swung by once more on my way out. There had been no change. 'I think you're safe to go home and get some sleep,' I suggested to Dad. 'We're just waiting for her to wake up now. I don't think anything is going to happen immediately.'

The following morning, I arrived to learn there had been no change overnight, so in that prediction I'd been right. I was beginning to worry that there should have been more progress, though. I spoke with the ICU doctor and the anaesthetist, and we discussed reducing the sedation levels further. The next day there had still been no change. Now I was beginning to get concerned. I ordered another brain scan. It showed a much healthier scene. There seemed little reason for the girl to still be unconscious.

A week passed with no further developments. Two more scans confirmed an angry-looking brain – swollen and showing signs of injury from the initial terrible event – but, crucially, no deterioration. Again, it's not exactly something families are equipped to deal with.

'Well, at the moment what we do know is that your daughter hasn't got worse.' Yeah, that never gets the champagne corks popping.

Day eight came and went, and I fully feared that day nine would be the same. I was consulting on another case when my beeper went off. When I checked the call, I burst into the largest grin. It was news of my young coma patient. She hadn't suddenly leapt out of bed and started doing the can-can. She hadn't begun reciting the Greek alphabet. She hadn't demanded pizza and pop. She had, however, brought up her hand – which is what we call localizing – and moved when the nurse was adjusting her breathing tube.

On the face of it, what's a hand movement? But the family and nurses knew. It was the first thing that had emanated from the young patient – their young daughter, niece, granddaughter – in more than a week that wasn't the product of drugs or machinery. It is a very visceral human reaction to discomfort. The little lady was feeling something. She was waking up.

I was as pleased as anyone. All the important brain signals were beginning to spike into life. 'I think we're ready to bring her out,' I said. 'How long do you think it'll take to get her fully off the sedation?'

'Hopefully within forty-eight hours,' the anaesthetist said. 'We're going to take it slowly.'

The waking-up process for an adult, let alone a child after that time period, is a slow one. The ICU doctors and anaesthetists still need to okay the heart function. They're in charge, so I step back. Waiting and waiting, just like the family.

The next twenty-four hours were excruciating. We all hoped for another sign of consciousness and we were all disappointed. Had it been a one-off? Was it a glitch after all? Why had nothing else happened? I was actually on my rounds the following morning when the next sign materialized. And that sign was historic. She was fighting the tubes that were sticking out of her, anxious to sit up. In other words, being a terrible patient – and no one could be happier. Distress at the tube in her throat indicated that she was able to breathe unaided. She was drowsy, but awake and engaged. Within another three days she was eating and speaking.

I have to say, Mum and Dad could not thank me enough. They spoke of me in front of their daughter as though I was someone just between Santa Claus and God. Now, I am well aware that in real life I am probably somewhere between Mr Greedy and Mr Grumpy, but still I would be lying if I said that we don't love getting compliments. We don't believe them, sure, but these positives are what we stash away to tide us over the next, inevitable, dark time around the corner. The truth is, that little darling on the bed didn't know me from Adam. She had no idea I'd touched her brain. No idea of anything, in fact, since her collapse a fortnight earlier.

I was happy to leave it that way. After everything she had been through why burden her with unnecessary information? She'd discover who I was soon enough when she came back for us to remove the AVM problem once and for all. Until then, however, I was happy just being another random grown-up.

CHAPTER ELEVEN

CSI OXFORD

Golf can be very dangerous for your health. Depending on the company, that is.

During my time in Glasgow I came to recognize the differences between a driver, an iron and a putter. Not from playing the game or even watching it on TV. I really had very little interest in those days, preferring bars and parties. No, back then my entire knowledge of golf clubs stemmed from identifying the telltale impression that each one left when it was smacked into a person's head.

It was the start of an interesting sideline to my day-to-day job – giving medicolegal advice to courts and investigations involving neurosurgical areas of expertise. I've been called upon more than once to give expert evidence in court about weapons used for assault or murder. Golf clubs are reasonably easy to identify. They leave a certain distinctive blunt trauma site in the scalp, skull and brain. Other implements require a little more investigation.

I was once called upon to look over evidence from a particularly nasty torture and murder in Newcastle. Four men had been arrested. CCTV showed them all attacking the victim, but each of them was wielding a different type of weapon: one had a hammer, one an axe, one a samurai sword, of all things, and one had a knife. The question was: which one had delivered the fatal blow?

Without a single person to accuse, there was a strong possibility that all four men would get off the murder charge. At least that was the angle the defence teams were playing. If the prosecution didn't realistically think that they could prove which of the group was the one responsible, then there was apparently no way they could prosecute successfully to the level they wanted to.

I was called in to provide some thoughts. Very clearly all four weapons had played their part in the victim's horrific last moments. The broken bones in the arms were caused by the hammer. The missing fingers were consistent with the sharp blade of the samurai sword. As for what had caused the massive damage to the head, however, that was unclear. Photographic evidence suggested it could have been the hammer or the handle of the sword or the back of the axe. The problem was, the head was so damaged in places that it was impossible to get a reading on what had gone on. Which is where my new toy came in.

I have special software which I can use to feed in the scans and reconstruct the original skull and brain shape. At the time, it was not widely used, although of course technology moves forward rapidly and now it's quite standard practice. It was very *CSI Oxford* for its day. I was able to 'rebuild' the skull and brain at the point of injury. I found a very clear trauma tract in the skull and brain caused by a single blow consistent with the size, shape and weight of ... the hammer. It fitted very well with the opinion of the pathologist who did the post-mortem. In such cases, it is really helpful to have different sorts of evidence that all agree – thus minimizing the risk of making a mistake with the medical interpretations.

Sometimes I just review evidence remotely and provide a paper report – especially if my evidence contributes to a decision not to move forward with an investigation. If there is a case to answer, often I 'appear' in court via a video link. Other times I go in person. Most barristers think that juries respond better to 'real' people. Several cases, I think, have been dependent either way on my evidence. I think that I have developed the skills to address a court as a result of my day job. We have to explain medically complex conditions to very stressed families, so we get used to going slowly, using non-technical language and picking up on when things aren't clear to people unfamiliar with medical matters. You can see its effects ripple across the room as everyone thinks, 'Yeah, I understand now.'

Case in point: a student in Manchester had the misfortune to get into altercations twice in one night. Again, pub cameras caught both incidents. You can clearly see him being punched around 8 p.m. and then again about 10 p.m. by a different person in a different bar. Only the second time he didn't get up.

The second attacker was charged with murder. His defence asserted that the punch wasn't hard enough to be fatal and that it was the earlier fracas which had 'triggered' the death. It was a persuasive argument. Certainly one to cause 'reasonable doubt' when considering the severity of the charge. I could see it written on the jurors' faces.

I was able to show that, from the scans, the victim had sizable areas of trauma. There was no way, I said, that he could have functioned if these had been caused by the first blow. No way he could have walked into the next pub, let alone ordered and drunk a beer.

As I delivered my evidence, I could see and feel the jury listening. By the time I had concluded that it was indeed the second event which was responsible for the killer blow, I think I had all twelve men and women either understanding why I believed that, if not agreeing with me.

Of course, when giving evidence, I am not trying to win a case. That's the job for the barristers. I am there to give the medical facts and then my opinion about what happened. After that, it's all down to the jury and the court.

Another week, another case. I was asked to investigate a mugging that had apparently got out of hand. Two men had been found with the victim's belongings. While they weren't denying assault and theft, they completely swore that the murder wasn't on them. 'Oh yes, we punched him and took his phone, but that was it. Someone else must have killed him.'

Interestingly, the evidence from the scans supported their version of events. While the victim had a bleed on the surface of the brain, he didn't have any kind of external signs of injury on that side of the head at all. The only oddity was a tiny little puncture wound on the opposite side.

The post-mortem report gave no further help. It cited a brain problem as cause of death, but stated it was very difficult to narrow down what actually was the weapon or method that was involved. Something wasn't right.

I reconstructed the scan using my 3D system. Once it was complete, I found I could draw a line from the very small puncture wound on one side of the head through the brain to the injury on the other side. En route, the line passed a very important artery – now bisected. Clearly that was the cause of death. This tract was not visible on the scans when he was brought in, and obviously the treating doctors weren't involved in the investigation. By the time the post-mortem was done, the brain tract had collapsed and disintegrated to a point where it could not be followed through the gelatinous, partially destroyed brain. However, the line of trauma became visible when I altered all the angles of the slices of the scans. Now it was a matter of the police proving how this had happened.

I advised the police to look for a certain shape of object. I predicted they'd find something like a narrow knife or another implement with a fine blade. In the end, they discovered a very thin 6-inch screwdriver in a bin. Basically, it turned out that the aggressors had meant to threaten the victim, but he'd fought back and the tool had gone into his head. Clearly with some force, but it had been clean. One puncture straight in, straight out. Not only had it passed through the skull, but also the brain. The tragedy was that it had gone all the way through with minimal damage – but had just nicked a blood vessel on the other side.

To be fair, the post-mortem had discovered the entry point, but with the blood vessel on the other side of the brain the pathologist hadn't spotted the connection. Neither had I – it just slowly became visible as I played with the scans, turning them around on the screen. I had a long chat to the pathologist afterwards and we talked about how independent but confluent bits of work had come together so well. This is an important thing to bear in mind as cost cutting continues to affect both NHS and legal services in the UK.

◆

Playing Poirot is all well and good, but my main specialism, the thing I'm most known for in medicolegal fields, is something far more tricky. As a paediatric neurosurgeon, the medicolegal cases I'm going to see are never nice.

There is a difference between medicine and law. My job is not to say whether somebody's guilty or not guilty, but rather to explain what I think is the cause of death or likely cause of injury. I can say, 'This injury is consistent with a traumatic assault that took place between ten and twelve o'clock this morning.' If that timing happens to narrow down the number of suspects, then all the better for justice, but that's not why I'm there. In fact, equally important is looking for any medical or 'innocent' causes or contributions to brain and spinal injuries.

The majority of cases involving children are heard at the Family Court. There's no jury, just a judge. Usually I'll appear via video link and I won't be the only expert witness. I have taken part in trials where there have been four or five of us on the stand together, chattering away, which is known as 'hot-tubbing'. More standard practice, however, is each of us giving evidence separately. It has the benefit of you not being swayed by the arguments of your colleagues.

I'm usually the only neurosurgical expert involved in a case. There's an eye expert, an X-ray expert and a general paediatric expert, all looking at the same evidence. It's paid work and it's interesting. Most of all, it's important. Currently, there are only a few paediatric neurosurgeons in the country doing this sort of thing – worries about being cross-examined or not wanting to read pretty unpleasant material or occasional disgruntlement about the legal aid board or CPS fees all serve to put medical professionals off this vital strand of medicolegal work.

If it's a case that's got as far as court, then you can imagine the degree of scrutiny that has already been levelled at the family and carers. There will be stories of previous histories of drug and alcohol abuse, domestic violence and even injuries sustained by other children in the family. I can't get invested in that, though. Although statistics suggest that such circumstances may make it more likely that a person would commit an offence, it doesn't prove it medically, in terms of the actual injury I am looking at. Otherwise we could just decide that once you have a criminal past you will be guilty of any charge brought against you. Guilt or innocence is for the judge and jury to decide. As soon as you start getting involved in the emotional side of it, you've lost your position as an independent witness and expert.

Luckily, there's a lot of good material available these days to help us. A doctor in Germany in the 1980s conducted some incredible research into this area. Somehow he obtained permission from the parents of recently deceased babies to allow him to 'experiment' on their bodies, which involved dropping them from different heights in order to measure the level and area of fractures on the skull. Through his work, he showed that babies could sustain a fracture from a fall from a much lower height than had been previously thought. It sounds an absolutely grotesque way to conduct medical research, but not only was it legitimate and correctly organized, I'm convinced that its findings have been used to help prove the innocence or guilt of hundreds of people in these sorts of cases. One wonders if the parents know the difference their babies have made in this field, and whether that may give them some comfort.

• • ✦ • •

It's such a common occurrence, sadly. This is just one story. It begins with a woman and a baby – although technically the woman is really still a child. She has a boyfriend who is not the baby's father. He comes and goes, doesn't help around the house and resents the baby interfering with his sex life. Much of his time is spent smoking skunk and drinking. Eventually, Mum persuades him to look after Baby for a couple of hours while she goes out with the girls for the first time since the birth. She's looking forward it. So desperate for a change of scene that she maybe ignores the warning signs.

While the mother is out the baby is, quote unquote, being played with when it suddenly collapses, goes into a respiratory arrest – it stops breathing and clearly becomes exceedingly unwell. An ambulance is called, Baby is taken to hospital and found to have a variety of intracranial injuries – bleeding on the surface of the brain and injury within the substance of the brain itself. There is blood in the spine as well. The ophthalmologists look and find bleeding behind the eyes. They state that these are clear evidence of injuries. There are long bone injuries to the limbs, and multiple ages of rib fractures.

By the time the notes of the case are passed to me, many other people have come to their conclusions. I'm not interested in those. I'm being paid for my expertise as a neurosurgeon, not my ability to parrot someone else's opinion. It's clear that the treating doctors think this child has experienced a recent traumatic event on a background of old abusive events. They believe that this one was not just 'out of the blue'.

Not everyone who looks dodgy is dodgy. And even those who are dodgy aren't necessarily child abusers. So what I can't do is blame a specific person. What I can say is that this baby suffered a traumatic event after being seen looking perfectly well by three different people at 8 p.m. on the evening in question. It's then up to the police and Crown Prosecution Service, or the Family Court to decide a) whether my evidence is correct and b) whether it indicates a particular suspect.

The defence's case, such as it is, is that Baby fell. My initial response is that two-month-old children have zero ability to climb. Even if they did fall, however, a careful comparison of the findings in this case with the medical literature built up over a century, and my clinical experience built up over somewhat less than that, shows a massive difference between probable injuries as a result of a fall from a sofa height compared to the actual injuries.

I complete my observations and post them back to the court. The event occurred in September. I've been instructed and reported some six months later in March. The trial begins in August.

Later in the year I give my evidence online. It is consistent with other evidence and the jury finds that the partner injured the child. In my heart and mind I am confident it's the correct decision based on the facts I've read. Which is why, eight months later, I'm so surprised to see that he has won an appeal. I am told that it's on a 'legal technicality' rather than a point of medical evidence.

But it's irrelevant: it doesn't help the baby, now facing a life of major neurological injury and disability. But this is how it must happen – it's a legal process that has run alongside the treatment and rehabilitation of a small child whose brain function will never recover to any significant level. Feeding tube insertion to the stomach, blindness, lack of voluntary movement or speech – this child's life, and his mother's, has been massively and irrevocably changed. Justice, I muse, is at least something we can offer them.

◆ ◆ ◆ ◆ ◆

I've written around 500 reports for court cases over fifteen years. I've even got some of my other consultant colleagues interested in working in this area now, just as Peter had encouraged me. What I tell everyone, though, is that you can't be on the side of the defence or the prosecution, of the victim or the family or the accused. You have to just follow the evidence and present it in as coherent a manner as possible. Even if no one else agrees.

I was called in on a case involving a carer accused of striking a baby with enough force to kill her. The carer insisted that she'd done nothing wrong. All she could state is that Baby had died from injuries sustained after falling from the changing table. However, because that had happened twenty-four hours earlier – in front of a witness – it was ruled out as a potential cause of death, which left the woman fighting to prove her innocence.

In this case there were no historical injuries to Baby. Just one area of impact trauma on the brain. The falling story seemed plausible. Except for the time at which it occurred. The prosecution had the testimony of four eminent experts in the field. Since death was recorded during the time that the carer was alone with the child, they all concurred that the time when the baby collapsed was the time of the trauma. 'Babies don't just go off in your hand', I read in one report.

I was aware of a single case report by a couple of pathologists in New York which discussed a nine-month-old baby who had fallen off a bed and seventy-two hours later, having apparently been well in between, was found dead. The post-mortem showed fracture and a brain injury as cause. That the child had been fine for seventy-two hours after the fall shows that, however rare, it was certainly possible for a child to have an impact injury and then have a so-called lucid interval, when they can behave normally, before becoming very unwell or worse.

The problem of being the first person to discover something is that nobody's ever heard of it before, so the New York case attracted much attention. Everybody in the US who investigated couldn't find any evidence of abuse except for the bumps caused by falling out of bed – which had happened in front of a relative. It was then written up as a 'fatal delayed complication of an impact injury'. I found it very interesting and wondered whether I was looking at another case of it.

Because of the controversial nature of my report, I was asked to attend court in person. I had already handed over the article to my instruction team, but they weren't under any obligation to give it to the prosecution.

When the prosecution's first expert witness came out, I felt challenged. I hadn't been doing expert witness work long, and he sounded very knowledgeable. He wasn't having any of my theory. The defence then asked him whether he had read the case report.

'No.'

'Another copy, please?' the defence barrister asked the clerk of the court.

And so it went for three more experts. Only one of them had read it – and I am not sure if that was beforehand or while he was waiting in court watching the others being cross-examined. And at the end they all had the same answer. While they thought it unlikely that a child could be injured, then a day later succumb to those injuries fatally, they had to admit it was possible. And that offered reasonable doubt to the defence.

The jury were actually saved from making a decision by the prosecution counsel, who stood up and announced that they were withdrawing the charge.

I was pleased with the outcome, and not just because I had been a lone voice in the defence. There was only one child in the paper published, but it didn't matter. It proved there was sometimes no black and white in these cases. But it still meant that it was a very unlikely event, leading me to consider whether it was more likely that a different cause was behind it all – maybe one involving abuse?

What would have happened if that same carer had been accused of another identical assault six months later? Of course, I would mourn any baby's illness or death – even more so in these circumstances. But I have to take a leaf out of the barrister's book. They operate a taxi-rank system – take the next case that comes along, regardless of which side it's for. I do the same. Defence, prosecution, family – it is all the same to me. It has to be to avoid becoming a biased 'hired gun'. I tell myself that I have to follow my training. I'm a paediatric neurosurgeon. That's my area of expertise. Stick to the facts. It is for others to interpret the law. But still, what if?

All this worry and self-doubt chips away at you, but I have to remember just what is at stake here, both for the defendant and for the tiny victim. And if it is a parent under suspicion or on trial, how much worse must it be if you know you are innocent and aren't even afforded the time and space to mourn or look after your baby?

CHAPTER TWELVE

SUCK IT AND SEE

No patient is ever really done and dusted. At least, that's how we in paediatric neurosurgery see it. Anyone that passes through our doors is rarely more than six months or a year from returning for a check-up. It doesn't matter what you came in for or in what condition you leave, there could be years of assessment before the full discharge notice is signed. Just because we've fixed one thing, it doesn't mean it can't cause other symptoms elsewhere in the body. Some brain conditions happen overnight. Others build up undetected for years before the diagnosis is made.

Many of the days when I'm not operating are spent dealing with outpatients in clinic or the day ward. I love it. It's such a potpourri. Children can alter immeasurably in a year. Each time I step out into the waiting room and call a name, I have no idea which person is going to come forward – the cute little pigtailed girl from last year is now heavily made-up, complete with Goth outfit. She is still adorable, but I can't say that to her now!

In theory, every operation we perform is intended to leave the patient in a better condition than before, or at least stop the situation worsening. Surgery is a big risk. I'd never do it unless there was a chance of success. Even the misjudgements arise from a desire to improve. The truth is, we can do everything right in theatre, achieve everything we set out to do, but we still don't know if it's successful until that patient wakes up. Even then it could be days, weeks or months before the benefits are fully revealed. Or the drawbacks. The truth is, it's not always good news. And not everyone gets to walk away.

It's a clinic day. I've seen the list of patients due to attend their annual or bi-annual check-up. Most of them were mine originally and the ones whose faces I still remember. Others were operated on by my colleagues. What I don't know is what they'll be like when they arrive. I'm always excited to see.

'Clare?' I call out to the packed room. 'Clare Bennett?'

Let's rewind to three months earlier. I was referred this young girl, whom the paediatrican had diagnosed with a condition called Chiari malformation, an abnormality of the back of the base of the brain where tissue extends down into the spinal canal. She was seven when we first saw her and a lovelier young bundle of happiness you would be hard-pressed to find.

Chiari malformation can be completely asymptomatic – that is, cause absolutely no problems in a patient. Trouble is, in the next one it can be extremely debilitating. If the spinal cord is getting squashed it can affect the function in your arms and legs, with poor balance, pain or funny feelings in the limbs, and often reduced strength even in walking on the flat. It can also affect the nerves supplying the lower part of your face, so chewing or swallowing, plus speech and even eye function, can all be affected.

Clare was born with some mild cerebral palsy (CP), causing weakness in her left side.

Chance had played a sneaky hand in Clare's treatment. As she grew and struggled with walking and hand function, her parents and doctors, naturally, put everything down to her CP – this is what CP causes. It was only around the age of six or seven when it became obvious that she was suffering in both sides of her body, not just on her weaker left side, that someone said, 'We'd better do a scan here to see what's going on.' They were expecting to see more problems in the brain, where CP causes its changes, but actually they found an abnormality in what we call the craniocervical junction, the crossing between the brain and the spine.

By the time she was referred to me, Clare had deteriorated further, with wobbly hand function, lots of headaches, and really struggling to walk. She was in a right state and getting progressively worse according to notes from her referring doctor. That, as I told her and her parents, was what we had to address.

'I think we need to operate,' I said to all three of them.

'Can you fix me, Doctor Jay?' Clare asked.

'Maybe,' I said. 'But the main thing is to stop things from getting worse.'

I explained how the condition could exacerbate over time. The classical teaching is that the aim of surgery here is to stop a deterioration. So we tell the patient, 'We can't get back what's already been lost. But we can protect the rest – the function you still have.'

Secretly, though, I hoped for more. The body has a way of healing in these cases. I wouldn't have been surprised to see some motor function return within months. We have tended to operate earlier in the disease history than many units, and we have noticed a proportion of patients get a recovery and regain some of the lost function. But since it would be a bonus – and we couldn't predict which patients would get the recovery, I don't offer that up for the family – it wouldn't be fair to make a decision on that basis.

There are various ways of treating Chiari malformation. Like all surgeries they come with risks. In this case there was stroke and paralysis, breathing and swallowing problems, meningitis, death, and a risk that the operation doesn't work or has to be repeated – all of which I explained to Clare and her parents, but I got the thumbs up anyway. The majority of Chiari malformations respond to decompression surgery, so that's what we did. To the sounds of The Stone Roses' self-titled debut album, I removed a small piece of bone from the base of Clare's skull and another from the top of her spine. I opened up the dura and buzzed away the bottom bit of the brain to give the spinal cord and the brainstem some space. The bits we attacked are the cerebellar tonsils, and unless you are a shark or similar, you don't absolutely need them – a bit like the tonsils at the back of your throat. I was hopeful it would take effect immediately, as brain fluid could flow unimpeded into the spinal cord now that pressure on the brain had been reduced.

Most children are pretty unwell after this procedure – the foramen magnum decompression – with nausea, vomiting and feeling seasick, and in pain, for about seven days and it can take up to six months to get fully back to their preoperative state. But this time, the day following the operation, I was amazed to see that my young patient was not only awake but also back to her usual smiley self.

'Did you do it, Doctor Jay?' she asked, before I could get a word in. 'Did it work?'

'We did what we set out to do,' I said. 'Fingers crossed it worked.'

'When will we know?' Mum asked.

'Hard to say. I'm confident we've addressed the actual problem, if you like, so Clare shouldn't get any worse. But she's going to take time to actually mend from the operation, that could take weeks or months. You'll know before I do.'

I was really hoping for a recovery. It would not happen today or tomorrow or even next month, but I was thinking that it could come in part or in full eventually. We sent her home to recover from the operation, wobbly, but walking on her own. The question was, would she also recover from the Chiari itself?

And now, three months later in clinic, I was about to find out.

· · ✦ · ·

'Clare?' I call again.

I'm on the verge of returning to my clinic room, thinking, how unusual it was that she had DNA'd – 'Did Not Attend' – when I spy movement at the back of the waiting area. There's a bit of a kerfuffle as someone on crutches struggles to their feet. They don't quite have the strength to support themselves on their arms. I'm about to offer to help when I realize. It's her. It's Clare. *What the hell has happened*?

The whole family are as delightful as always. They're as mystified as I am as to why Clare has continued to deteriorate. Usually my clinics are for chatting and learning more than 'doing', but I am desperate to find some answers.

'Do you mind if we take some more scans, Clare?' I ask. 'It's possible that I didn't fully release the area during the last operation, or that things have scarred back up.' Both of these are potential causes of an ongoing problem. So I send her off for some urgent scans and book another clinic visit.

I wish it helps. But it doesn't. Everything on the scan looks exactly as I'd hope – there was loads of space around the brain now. So why is she getting worse? Another textbook operation with an unfathomable outcome. I sit there for a minute, my fingers pressed together in the 'church' pose. I'm thinking. Thinking and thinking.

'All I can suggest,' I say eventually, 'is that we have another go.'

All three of them – Mum, Dad and Clare – jump at the idea. For all their positivity, I think they are in dire need of a 'quick fix'. I need to temper this straight away.

'The facts of the matter are that we performed a good operation that should have gone a long way to stabilizing you. That hasn't happened. The scans look clear, but maybe there's something "invisible" to the scan that's in the base of your skull and doesn't want to go away – some small strands of scar tissue that are holding everything down, but which are too fine to see on the MRI. I would like another chance at finding it, but you should be aware of the risks.'

I trot them out: damage to the spinal cord, damage to the brainstem, damage to the brain, contraction of meningitis or some other serious disease.

Dad shrugs. 'Paracetamol comes with worse warnings.' I smile ruefully. Although this may be true, the fact is that the risks of a reoperation are almost always more than the first one, because we don't have the usual anatomical markers and layers to guide us.

'What would you do if it were your daughter, Doctor Jay?' Clare asks.

I think of my three girls sitting at home. 'You know what? I'd go for it. Yes, I don't know what I'm looking for. Yes, it's basically a fishing expedition. A suck-it-and-see mission. But given what's happened, I can't see an alternative, other than to accept that the deterioration *may* progress to paralysis.'

We perform the surgery. As predicted, it's more difficult the second time round. I wanted to double-check that the spine didn't need untethering, that there was free-flowing fluid and that the mobility of the skull and spine weren't being impeded or impacting on crucial nerves. But I find nothing. Zero. Squat.

The best I could do was to retrace my original footsteps and 'redo' the cuts I'd made. Perhaps we'd get lucky. That was the stage we were at. Calling on good fortune to dig us out.

Once again, I am surprised by just how ebullient Clare is in recovery. Her eyes sparkled with the joys of life. If I could have played the Joker card on anyone's health, I'm pretty sure I would have chosen her. She deserved it.

I report back to the family and confirm, once again, that all we can do now is wait. 'How long?' Mum asks.

'Let's say three months,' I reply. 'I really hope we'll see changes by then.'

And I was right …

• • ◆ • •

'Clare? Clare Bennett?'

It's the moment of truth. Nearly four months have in fact passed since I performed the second operation on the young girl with Chiari malformation and CP complications. I can't pretend that I thought about her every day – impossible given the number of people I treat each week – but she's not been far from my mind. More than anything I just want to know how she's doing.

I look around the waiting room. It's not so packed this time. Clare has the first appointment. I scan the closest faces. Listen for the kerfuffle of rubber stoppers being deployed on the shiny NHS floor. I hear nothing and for a second I'm pleased. It would make my day if Clare arrives without crutches.

She does. So why am I not smiling?

The double doors at the back of the room swing open and in comes my patient and her doting parents. Dad is pushing the wheelchair.

I really hope I manage to look as pleased to see them as they do to see me. Inside I'm in turmoil. What the hell has happened? When I first met Clare she was walking, albeit with a struggle. The second time, after my first intervention, she needed crutches. Now, after the operation that was meant to reverse the original misfortune, she can't even do that. She's in a wheelchair. What on earth is going on? *What have I done?*

• • ◆ • •

Fast-forward ten years and Clare is no longer in her chair. She can walk short distances and has mastery over her hands for the most part. And she's still smiling – with good reason. She is now a proud mother herself. Since turning eighteen she passed to the care of my colleagues in the adult section of the hospital. To this day I can't honestly say why she didn't respond to the treatment. It was textbook, the same process I've done many, many times with solid results. Nothing on her scans or her charts indicated anything out of the ordinary. And yet there she was. Getting worse and worse and worse.

You feel so powerless in these situations. I consulted with everyone I knew. No one could spot a flaw in the surgical treatment. The failing was somewhere between modern medical knowledge and Clare's personal DNA. My colleagues used the same platitudes that I offer them in other cases – 'life sucks sometimes', 'remember it's not you, it's the disease causing this', and 'you can't fix everyone'. They are right, of course, which is why we take so much time to consent before operating. Still, it doesn't help very much.

At least in her case I was able to try. At least when she'd first arrived I hadn't had to say 'Sorry, there's nothing I can do.' Because, trust me, that feels a damn sight worse.

CHAPTER THIRTEEN

MY LAST PATIENT DID REALLY TERRIBLY

Patients presenting similar symptoms can have wildly different causes. A child suffering from a sudden loss of leg function can be the result of a blood clot or a stroke. It can also be due to a tumour. Or it can be multiple sclerosis.

Many children who arrive with a bleed from a vascular malformation in the spinal cord don't get significantly better. Unsurprising odds, I'd say, for a condition that sees sudden rupturing of abnormal vessels which then spurt blood, under pressure, into the spinal-cord tissue itself. These are children who have been absolutely fine until the moment they're not. One minute they're haring around the house or their school and suddenly they drop to the floor with total loss of leg function. No warning. Complete paralysis. They're taken to hospital and a massive blood clot is discovered in the spinal cord.

It's not often you find yourself hoping for a tumour, but sometimes it can prove to be the least worst option. Loss of leg function caused by tumorous clot is attackable. We can operate.

Go in, get the bastard, retreat. Job done. Vascular or blood vessel problems sound less terrifying, but they're harder to put right.

If you think about it, whatever blood vessel has ruptured, the clot has to some extent been contained by the fact that it's held within the spinal column, compressing the cord. Hence the loss of lower-limb function. It sounds obvious to try to unblock the passageway, but if you do, as well as being accurate you also have to be quick. When you open up the spinal dura, you're essentially opening the very structure that is containing this vascular malformation. All the blood vessels can swell out of control in front of you in a very tight, narrow space. Suddenly, the cord is being pushed out of the dural opening, and precious, vital nerve tissue is coming out, and you have to apply pressure to hold it in, but without damaging the spinal cord any further. In short, the situation can quickly turn into a disaster if you aren't careful. And that's being optimistic.

The current thinking with this type of problem, with the attendant risks of operating, is often very much 'let's wait and see', unless there is active deterioration in function. In other words, we're trusting in luck and our old friend, time.

The decision-making in these scenarios is about probabilities. About cause and effect. On the one hand, what are the chances that if you go in and remove this blood clot you will recover leg function? On the other, what are the chances that this is a very abnormal collection of blood vessels and so any surgical procedure may set off a tsunami of reactions with the haemorrhage spreading higher up the cord. In trying to save the knees, you could risk the hips. In trying to save the hips, you could put the upper torso at risk.

It sounds doom and gloom, but it's not always. If a local hospital says they've got a child with incomplete loss of function and it's been around four hours, there's still enough time for you to potentially save some function. Once there's been twelve hours of absolutely no function, your window of opportunity is beginning to close.

There's an element of chance. Some parents won't dial 999 until a leg actually falls off. They come from that stock of people who don't want to 'trouble' the emergency services. Their child starts falling over? They pack him off to bed with some Calpol and assume everything will be okay in the morning. Or maybe something happens during the night while the boy's asleep. Next day, Mum just thinks he's too lazy to get up, especially if it's a weekend.

Any number of reasons can delay a patient getting to hospital. Once there, the dice need to be rolled again. A lot of children's departments have very good A&E set-ups. Even so, it can be a decent amount of time before you get in front of the person with the authority to say, 'We need a scan.'

Or maybe they don't do that. Maybe they jump straight on the phone to their local specialist hospital. The John Radcliffe has one of the twenty or so stand-alone paediatric neurosurgical departments in the country. Where potential loss of function in children is concerned, it's our policy to have them shipped over immediately – we need to see them and ensure the information on which we are making such major decisions is accurate. I can't vouch for the way that other departments are run – I know from my medicolegal work that not all of the units around the country do this. So there's another element of chance based on geography. And all of it depends on another condition: the clock.

· · ◆ · ·

My phone rings one day. 'Jay, we've got incoming.'

'Who? What? Where?'

'Five-year-old boy, loss of leg function, day before yesterday. No scans done. Northampton rerouted straight here.'

'Okay, get him magnetized as soon as he arrives.' I tend to make up a lot of stupid words – this was my way of asking for an MRI scan.

The problem with a patient coming in 'hot' like this is that we're blind. The time element is worrying. Two days is a long time to have these sorts of symptoms.

The boy arrives with his parents. A registrar greets them and then gets the scans done. He's already had a look by the time he hands them over to me.

'What do you think?' I ask.

'Not good.'

'Yes, thanks, Doctor House! What else?'

'I don't think it's a tumour. The history seems wrong for that – either a vascular lesion or of course it could be a bleed into a tumour. It's a bit too fast for something like demyelination.' The latter term refers to a condition like multiple sclerosis, which can present similarly but has a very different treatment.

'How long since he's been well?'

'Maybe thirty-six hours.'

I pause. 'I fear the horse may have bolted.' But I don't tell the family that. Not yet. Not till I have all the information. Naturally, they're beside themselves.

'We're so sorry, we didn't realize it was so serious,' Mum sobs. 'I thought he was playing up.' Another common phrase where children are concerned. What kid hasn't feigned injury at some point for attention or to get out of chores or just for a laugh? Navigating the mindset of a young boy or girl can be a minefield for parents.

'It's not your fault,' I say. 'You didn't cause this.' Not directly anyway. Perhaps there's a genetic link. I run through a few questions. I want to know the family history, who's had what. It will help to narrow down the likely causes. Neither Mum nor Dad can offer any magic pointers from their family lines.

'What do you think it is?' Dad asks.

'It appears your son has a blood clot in his spinal cord caused by a burst vessel. The pressure has shut off power to everything south of that spot. Like a roadblock on the motorway. Nothing can get past.'

'Will he be all right? Can you cure him?'

That word again. My instinctive response is to recall the last chap I had in suffering from the same condition. I was too late to help then.

In his own sweet time, over the course of nearly twelve months, he started recovering, but only a bit. But I can hardly tell this family that 'my last patient did really terribly'. How's that going to help them?

What I can do – and what I will do – is to give them some hope. Positivity can go a long way to aiding or prompting recovery. There are numerous studies written about it. I want the parents to believe that there is a chance their boy can recover. And I need him to believe it, too. So I tell them about the body's natural healing qualities. How it can, over time, fix little glitches. Little glitches that have massive repercussions.

'Are you saying that you can't do anything at all?' Mum asks.

'I have to be honest with you. I don't know if we'll ever be able to get back to square one. But our best bet is to just wait and let nature take its course. We're going to run some more tests, but I'm afraid any operation we might try to do runs a high risk of making things worse.'

'Worse?' Mum says. 'Worse than not being able to walk? What's worse than that?'

The fact that so much time has passed gives clarity to my thoughts. If the collapse had happened just a few hours ago, I'd have a ton of quick decisions to make: 'Do I think I can help? Is the situation likely to deteriorate if I don't act? Is there a chance that, in trying to help, I'm going to make things worse?' And finally: 'Can an operation in this area be safely performed on a child of this size?'

The time that has elapsed means none of those questions are viable any more. The moment has passed. Pandora's box is open.

I look at the little guy tucked up in bed. You're on your own now ...

Size matters. If you stand on a full-flowing hosepipe in the garden, then take your foot off it, the build-up of water comes shooting out at top speed for a second, then settles back to normal flow. What doesn't happen is that you run out of water. That's because there's a considerable supply in the local water pipes, enough to cope with such shenanigans for hours, days and weeks.

A human body has a finite amount of blood. The average adult woman carries around 8 pints inside her. A man, depending on size, can have anything up to 10 pints or just over 5 litres. Children obviously have less, again dependent on size. By the time you get down to babies, you're looking at tiny amounts. At a few months old, a baby's blood volume will be between 250 ml to 350 ml – somewhere between a large glass of wine and a can of Coke. They don't have much to spare.

Any operation runs the risk of blood loss, but vascular difficulties, blood clots and the like are trebly dangerous. If a surgeon goes flying in looking for a clot, just disturbing it can cause the vessel to start spraying, especially an artery carrying oxygenated blood from the heart. It takes seconds for a baby to lose a harmful amount and not much longer for it to be devastating. A small five-year-old would also bleed out in a dangerously quick time. So you have to weigh up the desire to treat with the potential to actually make things worse.

As a general surgeon you wouldn't go in and tackle a vascular malformation in the liver if the whole organ is involved. But you may take the risk if there's just a small portion affected. You might say, 'We're going to cut out this bit of the lung' or 'We're going to remove this section of bowel with the vascular changes in it' – all perfectly sensible. Whatever it throws up should be manageable. But would you say, 'We'll take a piece of spinal cord?' knowing that rapid blood loss could make things go south very, very quickly? Probably not. Not on a child. Not unless there were no other options.

And that's without the normal problems associated with removing any part of the central nervous system. The long and the short of it is that you don't mess with anything hot and vascular unless you have a reasonably good shot at success. And with this kid, I didn't.

I've never felt so impotent. I'm a consultant at one of Britain's best paediatric neurosurgical hospitals (we think). I have resources that many units in other countries can only dream of. I have access to some of the greatest minds in the profession. But at the end of the day, we're all limited by science and physiology. Until someone devises a treatment for this condition, we just watch and we wait. And we hate every minute.

· · ◆ · ·

It's eighteen months later. I'm having a good clinic so far. Everyone I've seen since lunch has shown massive improvements since the last time they were here. There are few sights more life-affirming than families who believe they've been given a second chance. It's almost as though they've had a religious epiphany and seen the light.

The next name on my list is the young boy with the loss of leg function from a year and a half earlier. I remember when they were discharged. For every positive word that came out of my mouth, one of the parents countered it with some shrugged negativity. Even young Clare Bennett would have struggled to keep her countenance in their company. They didn't mean to, of course. They were in pain. Still blaming themselves and possibly each other for not acting sooner. And neither of them believed a word I'd said about time sorting everything out.

Their mood hasn't really improved in the interim. Or perhaps it has changed. They seem less angry and more resigned. Resigned to their lot. Resigned to their son being disabled for the rest of his life. Resigned to the fact that they think they could have done more.

I know they feel that *I* could have done more. They say it within the first few minutes. I reply how I always do: 'Most patients' bodies self-correct. It's still our best option. Surgery for this condition carries too many risks.'

For all the pain I can see the parents clearly suffering, the star of the show – the little fella who's actually suffering physically – just smiles at me. He's not blaming anyone.

'Mum, Dad,' he says. 'Stop arguing. I'm all right.'

I look at him and smile back. I offer my hand in the sort of clumsy fist bump that my daughters hate. 'Yes, big man,' I say. 'You are.'

CHAPTER FOURTEEN

SMASH A HOLE IN THE WINDOW

Who'd be a GP? You're having to deal with 64,000 different conditions from any site inside or outside the body, and every patient who comes in complaining of this pain or that may potentially have something that's about to go bang. What do you do? You can't send everybody to hospital for an urgent assessment even if you wanted to. It would bankrupt the NHS in an afternoon. You're a gatekeeper with your hands tied behind your back. So sometimes you have to make a call.

And sometimes you make a mistake.

· · ◆ · ·

A family went to see their GP with the general complaint that their three-month-old baby didn't seem quite right. 'Can you be more specific?' the GP asked.

'Well, he just doesn't seem to be like our other kids were.'

The GP had seen thousands of overcautious parents. 'Look, don't worry, every child is different. They all develop at their own pace.'

And so it went on. A month later the family returned. This time they were adamant. 'He doesn't move like the others did. He can barely turn his head.'

Once again the GP found nothing wrong, other than overanxious parents. And again he prescribed 'not to worry about it'.

You can picture the scene. I imagine this GP has probably just seen somebody with a heart condition beforehand, someone with a gammy leg prior to that and who knows what to come. He sees this child, he's got ten minutes to make an assessment, get a history off the family, do an examination, bang, bang, bang. Kiddie looks fine, he's probably okay, no obvious danger. But in this instance, there was. There really, really was.

Another fortnight passed by and the family had become seriously concerned. They knew they weren't making it up. This time they went to their local A&E. The doctor on call took one look at the boy and said, 'Blimey, he's got a big head' and then called in the paediatrician. Soon after, they were on their way to me. I took one look: 'Hydrocephalus.'

Hydrocephalus – from the Greek words meaning 'water' and 'head' – is a condition which sees a build-up of fluid in the brain, causing an increase in pressure in the head. In adults it can become serious quite quickly, as the brain pushes against the skull and has nowhere to go.

Diagnosing infants should – in theory – be a bit more straightforward. Because babies' skulls aren't fixed – they are basically a series of hovering plates that over time will fuse together – as their brains 'swell' they push the bones out and the entire head above the face balloons. On something as tiny as a baby, the difference in appearance can be extraordinary.

It's not the fluid itself that is the problem. All brains produce cerebrospinal fluid (CSF). It's necessary as a lubricant for the brain to sit in, like a kind of bath. Without it, every time you turned your head, your brain would bash against your skull like a tennis ball in a tin. It doesn't, though, because of the CSF.

The fluid is produced from the centre of the brain, sits in cavities called ventricles and is carried out via small exit holes. It runs down the spine and over the outer surface of the brain, gets reabsorbed back into the bloodstream and goes back to the heart as part of the blood. Production never stops. It's like a garden fountain, constantly recycling. It's a thing of beauty, really. Except when there is a blockage in one of the ventricles.

Hydrocephalus can be triggered by meningitis, tumours and occasionally have a genetic transmission. The majority of common or garden cases, though, come down to good old bad luck, plain and simple.

Everyone is born and for many of us the experience of delivery will prove so traumatic that the brain suffers a small bleed. Usually the blood will get reabsorbed by itself and won't leave behind any problems. In a small number of births, however, it may cause a clot and block the ventricle.

For all its wonderful potential, the brain can be remarkably unsophisticated at times. Block or no block, it carries on producing fluid like the Magic Porridge Pot, merrily ignorant that it is literally swimming in the stuff. It's the equivalent of pumping up an inner tube long after the tyre is hard. Hence the swelling. And the danger.

A decade ago, the family's concerns would have been picked up before the GP was even required to give an opinion. In the UK today, the circumference of a baby's head is measured at birth and again around the six-to-eight-week mark. It used to be the case that every time the health visitor called round, they'd measure the head and record it in the baby's 'little red book'. I don't know if it was to save money or part of yet another efficiency drive – probably both – but that is no longer standard practice. If it were, the little boy's condition could have been flagged earlier.

As it was, I had to surmise that his condition had set in after the eight-week reading, but that's not to say it wasn't caused at birth. The initial bleed can lead to a bit of scarring, which over time gets progressively worse until the passageway is fully obstructed.

The sad thing was, the clues were there. The baby not being able to lift his own head was the prime medical giveaway. Even before I was told this, there was a more obvious telltale sign. The baby's little T-shirt had a scissor cut around the neck.

'Your handiwork?' I asked the mum.

She nodded. 'I have to do that to all his tops. Otherwise I can't get his head through.'

I could have cried.

It's easy to knock the GP. I mean, babies *do* have large heads! And new parents *do* have a tendency to cry 'doom' at the sight of a cold. It's really easy for us specialists in our very rarefied, highly specialized field to be able to go, 'It's obvious, isn't it?' The truth is, heads and brains happen to be my area. If someone showed me a photo of a baby's foot and said, 'What do you reckon to this?' I'd go, 'I don't know, it looks like a foot.' Unless it was bigger or hairier than mine, or had six toes, I'm not sure I'd know what I was looking for.

Blaming anyone is never productive. All that mattered to that little baby and his parents was whether I could do anything about it.

I'd seen it so many times. Parents besides themselves with fear. The mere fact they'd been fast-tracked to see me after weeks of seeming indifference confirmed their worst nightmares, that things with their baby were serious. But they'd known that for a while. They had been the only ones. I just hoped they weren't blaming themselves.

'You're good parents,' I told them. 'You're experienced parents. You trusted your instincts and you didn't stop fighting even when you were assured there was nothing wrong. You did everything you could.'

I smiled. I wanted to put them at ease if at all possible. 'And now,' I said, 'it's my turn.'

Being told that there's something wrong with your child's brain must seem monstrously scary. And these two were terrified. It's not like learning little Johnny has sprained his ankle. The goings-on inside the head are unknown to most people. Beyond their ken. Sometimes it's beyond mine as well, but not this time. I explained about the probable little bleed, how common it is and how there was nothing they could have done to prevent it.

They took it all in, but then asked the question that everyone asks. 'Can you help him? Can you do anything? *Can you save our baby?*'

As I've said, one thing I will never do to parents or patients is lie to them. I won't tell them what they want to hear for the sake of it. It does no one any favours. It's rarely the easiest path and it certainly doesn't help me sleep at night. On this occasion, though, my candour wasn't going to be a problem.

'Hydrocephalus is a very serious condition and, let's be honest, it can look very unpleasant. However, there are procedures which we have successfully performed hundreds of times. I can't make any guarantees before we get into theatre, but there is a very strong chance that your son can be treated with this procedure.'

There was silence. There were tears. 'Thank you, Doctor Jay, thank you.'

Don't thank me yet – I haven't done anything.

There are two ways to surgically reverse hydrocephalus. One procedure has been around for sixty years. It's called a shunt – a tube that goes from head to abdomen, under the skin, and drains the excess fluid. In 50 per cent of cases further surgery is required within a couple of years. It's also linked to other complications including infection, which brings its own dangers. However, shunts have been used for a long time and, if needed, they work. Indeed, before they were invented, hydrocephalus was very often a death sentence, or at the very least would usually ruin the child's development.

The other option is newer, just a couple of decades old, and less invasive – if that's possible, considering you still have to enter the brain. It entails using a small endoscope, or fibre-optic pipe, to enter the ventricle and make a new drainage hole. It's only viable if the block is in certain locations, which for a lot of patients happens to be the case. In this instance we were fortunate. Scans provided the good news. The block was treatable from the top. We were going in.

⋅ ⋅ ◆ ⋅ ⋅

Another name for endoscopic treatment is MIS – minimally invasive surgery. At least that is always the hope. Essentially, I'll be inserting a tiny microscope into the middle of the baby's brain via a keyhole incision at the top of the head. Compared to a shunt the dangers, although rare, are very real.

I can see from the scans that the blockage is in an ultra-sensitive area. Not the sort of place where one can go poking around. For a start it has exquisite pain centres. It also governs eye control. Not only could an injury here leave the baby with a lifetime of pain or numbness, it could also result in him being unable to focus properly. Destroying the blockage, therefore, is a no-no.

I wait for my anaesthetist, Karen, to give me the nod. Nothing happens until she's convinced that the baby's safe. 'We're a go,' she says.

'Okay,' I reply. 'Could we have some music?' Once again, I have to have music – it helps me to concentrate, to focus. Not just in the operating theatre, but at my desk, in the car, when revising for exams. Basically, I would like music on whenever I am not asleep.

As the angry rhythmic chords of AC/DC's 'Thunderstruck' begin to ring out around the theatre, I incise the skin, line up the drill and enter the top of the baby's forehead. This is not the same as an adult drill. It's finer – so fine, in fact, that it would allow me, if I wanted, to remove the shell off an uncooked chicken egg.

I demonstrated this for the start of one of the TV documentaries our department was featured in, mostly because the producers refused to believe we can do this. They brought twelve eggs in a box to give me a real sense of how much they trusted me. Fortunately, I managed to do it on the first attempt – or they would have definitely got a good shot of me covered in egg white – whisked at 75,000 rpm …

It goes to plan. I glance at Karen's monitors. No change in the patient's condition. Time for stage two.

The endoscope is inserted into the expanded ventricle. Looking at my own screens I can make out the area of the blockage and the no-go zone. Just in front is another area surrounded by two really important structures: the pituitary gland (which controls the majority of hormones) and the basilar artery (a key blood-supply axis). It's also home to the mammillary bodies, which are responsible for memory. Again, not things you want to mess with.

Peter used to say to families: 'Imagine you're in a room filling with water. If you can't open the door, what do you do? Smash a hole in the window.' I pinched that off him and use it all the time now.

Between these super important structures I can see a 2-mm gap. If I am able to poke a hole through the middle – or 'smash the window' – it would give the fluid a new route out of the brain. That's the priority. Offer a diversion, break the dam and get the pressure down.

It sounds dangerous, and indeed it can be. So many things can go wrong. But I have the equipment and the experience. This operation was a huge deal back when I was a trainee and the procedure was in its relative infancy. My boss in Glasgow would set aside quite a long time and it was a bit of a palaver. As experience increased, hints and tips were collated worldwide and equipment was improved. It is now classed as 'routine' and can be done, from start to finish, in less than twenty minutes. Medical progress is amazing – it takes money, collegiate working around the world and often a pioneer to try what has never been tried before – but the outlook for patients just gets better and better for it.

As it is, the operation goes well, we make a small exit hole and get closed up with no worries. When I walk into the waiting room afterwards, I can see the torture behind the parents' eyes.

'We won't know for certain until up to six months have passed,' I say, 'but all indications are that the treatment has been successful.'

'Can we see him?'

'Of course. Follow me.'

· · ◆ · ·

Five years later, that little baby is now a little boy. A little boy with a proportionate-sized head and who gets cuter every time I see him. The pressure alleviation worked. The block is still there, but so is the diversion. I see him once a year for a check-up and he's never looked back, despite the best attempts of the Magic Porridge Pot.

If I had to guess, it's unlikely that we'll ever need to treat him again. The same can't be said for the other type of hydrocephalus treatment. That's not to say that we don't have an extremely high rate of success, it's just that in many cases it's not a permanent fix. Considering what's involved, perhaps it's not surprising.

One of my first cases of hydrocephalus was caught during the baby girl's six-week circumference check. In this instance, the parents had been completely unaware. They were first-timers, so everything was new and mysterious and rather frightening for them. The fact they'd suspected nothing made the diagnosis that little bit more painful to hear. The parents of the other child, as sad as they were about their baby's condition, were expecting worse news than we actually gave them. For these guys, it came out of the blue.

Still, the baby was in no obvious discomfort and appeared to be developing well. Very quickly, though, the scans showed that there was a problem with the final point of absorption of the fluid, and not a blockage along the pathway that could be circumvented.

I could smash all the windows I liked, but the fluid wouldn't be absorbed. Which meant going to Plan B.

· · ◆ · ·

To say that the shunt operation is twice the procedure is quite literally true. For a start it ideally uses two surgeons. While I'm concentrating on the top end, my colleague is prepping the tummy. Between us and the nurse we have to ensure the baby is positioned in such a way that I can reach the back of her head and the registrar has access to her abdomen.

With the all-clear from the anaesthetic end of the room we begin. Firstly, I have to get through the scalp. It's a standard 'horseshoe' cut – a large letter 'U' carved around the area I need – then carefully I peel back the skin. It's such a small flap of a thing even compared to a ten-year-old's, let alone to that of an adult. What's inside is even smaller.

I drill a small hole in the bone and open up the dura – the fibrous bag around the brain. Now for the tricky part. I feed a very fine silicone tube into the fluid space in the middle of the brain. That, if you like, is the pipe that's going to drain out the excess CSF. It needs to go straight in for 8 cm.

To aim the tube with the greatest accuracy, I have looked at the scans. These are 2D slices which I use to build up into a 3D model in my head. I then look for external landmarks – the entry into the ear, the inner and outer angles of the eye, the bridge and tip of the nose, and plot them on my internal model. With these pointers, I think about where I will place the initial incision, the entry hole in the skull and the opening onto the brain surface. Then I plot what precise direction I need to angle the tube at so that it goes through the least important brain structures possible and into the fluid spaces. Even then, it must go into the correct part of the ventricles, so that it is less likely to get blocked further down the line. It is one of the commonest procedures we do in neurosurgery, but also one that is fraught with difficulty. The list of potential problems with putting this tube into the fluid spaces is huge.

I have caused weakness on one side of the body when I missed some very small ventricles and ended up in the movement control centre. I have also caused small loss of visual field to a patient when my entry point created a small bleed. The passing of the tube, once through the outer surface of the brain that I can see, is essentially blind – there is simply no way of knowing if the tube will catch a small vessel on its way towards the ventricles. If that leads to bleeding in the brain, it can cause a stroke. If it bleeds into the ventricles, it can enable the shunt to block very rapidly or force the operation to be abandoned.

I call shunt insertion the great leveller – any neurosurgeon, of even the highest seniority, can have really major problems while inserting a shunt, though seemingly one of the simplest operations we do. It underlies the simple fact that we tell families when requesting their consent that there is no simple neurosurgery – it's all fraught with danger and risk. 'Now sign here, please.'

I cut a pocket under the skin I've peeled back. With care I can feed a metal tube into the tissue layer between the skin and the rest of the body down the baby. Think of the layer when a butcher is skinning a rabbit – there are no major vessels or structures that can be damaged, as long as I stay in the right place. It's all done by touch and instinct. I feed with one hand and feel the impression of the tube beneath the surface. Down the back of the neck, round the side, over the shoulder bone and over the ribcage. To anyone watching it's like a little mole burrowing just beneath the surface.

There are no maps, but I know where I mustn't go. I have to navigate over the sheath that contains the carotid artery and the jugular vein in the neck, and the lung in the chest. One snick of those could cause more problems than I'm attempting to solve.

The ultimate destination is the abdomen, which is where my colleague has been working. He seems on track. The small incision has been made in the tummy, so he's got access to the abdominal cavity.

'Everything okay?' I ask.

'Ready when you are.'

We can both see I'm close. Even so, when the breakthrough comes, when we see the end of the tube pop out where the tummy incision has been made, it's still a relief. It's not a long distance in real terms – less than 30 cm – but such a journey.

The plan is for the brain fluid to be reabsorbed by the bowel. What we mustn't do, however, is damage it in any way. The last thing we want is to open up a shuttle system for the baby's poo to reach the brain. The infection risk would be huge. The bowel, with all its lovely contents, sits in a bag. It's the bag we need to breach. Once the tube is inside, all the superfluous brain fluid can be fed in and dispersed naturally.

The tube I'm threading through is actually two tubes, one inside the other. I remove the inner one and the actual shunt is pushed, cajoled and occasionally suctioned down through the tunnel we've made. When it reaches the abdomen, we remove the outer tube. We're nearly there.

The shunt is connected to a valve. This is a mechanism of balls and springs – and precious jewels. At a certain pressure the valve will open to let the fluid escape. It's crucial that the little door never sticks or becomes infected or causes irritation. I don't know who discovered this, but it turns out that rubies make the ideal gateway for some designs, which is why, for many decades, most of the shunts for the world were made in Switzerland. The manufacturing companies poached lots of watchmakers to help build their shunts – almost everything was done by hand.

My colleague stitches the tummy. I make good the scalp. We're two hours into our day and, if I say so myself, it's been a good one so far.

I go out to meet the parents. I hate the idea of keeping people waiting for news. A single second in a hospital waiting room can seem like an eternity – as I know all too well.

* * ◆ * *

The pipe inside baby Julia almost certainly saved her life. Apart from a tiny bump on her neck, which you'd really have to search for to notice it, you'd never guess there was a tube running down inside her. Today, she no longer has the original one. Man-made objects just weren't meant to sit inside the human body forever. There's always a risk of infection, decay and irritation from the pipe. Sometimes they just go wrong – they can block or stop working properly, just like a TV or a car. But the good news is that they're fixable.

Julia and those like her will never be 'cured'. They'll always carry a little piece of silicone around inside them. But many will never really notice it. The shunt quietly works away, letting our patients live as near normal a life as possible.

CHAPTER FIFTEEN

WHAT WOULD YOU DO?

I recognized the obstetrician's voice as soon as I picked up the phone. It was rarely good news when he called, but I couldn't hold that against him.

'Jay, can you come over?' he said. 'I need you to take a look at something.'

'What have you got?'

'Spina bifida.'

'Okay,' I said. 'Can you send me the scans. Then I'll talk to the family.'

'We don't have scans,' the obstetrician replied.

'Then how do you know it's spina bifida?'

'Because I'm staring at the newborn baby right now – he's just been born!'

· · ✦ · ·

Spina bifida is a congenital defect, which means it develops while the baby is growing inside the mother. In severe cases, the skin, muscle and bone don't cover a section of the spinal cord, affecting nerve function everywhere below. It can occur anywhere along the spine and can be denoted by a very visible hole in the back, often surrounded by a raw-looking protuberance.

The effects vary depending on where the hole is located. As a general rule of thumb, the higher up the spinal column it is, the higher the anatomical level of function lost. If the abnormality is very low down in the spinal cord, it can affect the bladder and bowel, which are controlled by the lowest nerves to come off the spinal cord. Then maybe the ankles. As you go up the spine, it may then start to have a damaging effect on your hips, *as well as* your ankles, bladder and bowel. Once it starts affecting the hips, you're much less likely to be able to walk. You can have a lack of sensation and problems with sexual function. There can be associated brain disorders that impact upon swallowing, speech and breathing function. Many patients will need a shunt for associated hydrocephalus.

For some, all these potential problems may make them think that there is no good news. But lots of patients who have spina bifida go on to lead happy, fulfilling lives – albeit totally different ones to what their parents were expecting for them. And there is no getting away from the fact that the initial conversations with an expectant mother or couple are almost universally a pivotal controlling moment in that baby's future. Which is why we scan so carefully these days.

For a lot of new parents, the twenty-week ultrasound scan is the most exciting time after being told they're expecting. That's the moment that can reveal whether you're having a little Johnny or a little Jenny. Whether or not you want to be told the gender, who doesn't get a kick out of catching a first glimpse of those tucked-up legs, little nose and those tiny, tiny hands? But while Mum and Dad are thinking about whether to buy printouts or videos from the session, the sonographer's interest is more than cosmetic. They monitor the heartbeat, measure the spine and check where the placenta is sitting. Basically, ticking off the baby's development against forecasts. They're the gatekeepers. The first line of defence against possible anomalies. Which is why, you'd think, everyone would make it a priority to see them.

· · ◆ · ·

When I meet the parents, they are distraught. Stunned, silent, uncommunicative. Mum is in bed, recovering after giving birth. Dad is staring out of the window. He says 'hello' when the obstetrician introduces me, but his attention soon drifts back out towards the car park. It's clear that they've both been crying.

'You've been told your baby has what is known as spina bifida?' I say. Mum nods.

'And what it means?' Another nod.

'Usually, these things are picked up during the mid-term scan,' I say as gently as I can. 'But we have no records of that.'

'We didn't have one,' Mum replies.

'Okay. Do you mind if I ask why not?'

'We didn't think you had to.'

These wouldn't be the first young people who either couldn't be bothered or forgot. That's one view. Of course, it's possible that they didn't really understand how important the scan is. They're pregnant and they've had it confirmed, so life carries on. People have to work – and now there is additional financial pressure on the family. The mother may need to take time off both before and after delivery, so the father may be being super careful not to annoy his boss by asking for more days off, to avoid increasing the risk of being sacked. Medical appointments may seem less important when you face the possibility of not paying this month's rent. Ninety-nine times out of a hundred, nothing too drastic comes of missing an appointment or a scan. But occasionally things do go wrong, and, in the case of this young couple, they're left to pay a high price. Or rather, their baby is.

When I first got into neurosurgery, I swore I would treat the whole family as my patient. Where a child's relatives are concerned, adults and siblings can feel the pain as keenly as the little one in the incubator. Or so it seems to them. But every so often I get a reminder that there really is only one patient.

I discuss the whole situation with the family, going through the facts of the condition, treatment plans and risks. It's a hell of a lot to take in at once. Without turning from the window, Dad asks me if Baby is going to be all right. Can I 'fix' him?

'There is no magical cure,' I reply. 'We will do our very best to get the back closed and prevent any more risk of infection or worsening of leg and bowel function. But we can't get back what has already been damaged.'

· · ✦ · ·

The first, most urgent 'fix' for a spina bifida baby is to get the hole covered. Inside the mother they are protected by the amniotic fluid in the sac. The dangers begin from the moment of delivery. The vaginal canal is, to be blunt, a contaminated area and it only gets worse from there. Not only is the baby dragged out into the open and exposed to an alien atmosphere, it's arrived in a place where sick people congregate. Even the nicest, cleanest hospital is still a house of infection. So, the very first priority is to close that hole as quickly as we can. This is not about regaining any function that the baby may not have but is simply to keep meningitis and the other Big Bads from the door.

There's no point talking the talk if you can't back it up. For an open newborn spina bifida case I'd ideally want them in theatre within forty-eight at the latest. On this occasion, I cleared the schedule and we were in the next day – within twenty-four hours of birth. I say 'we' because I wouldn't be alone. A colleague from plastic surgery would be on hand to assist.

There are several types of spina bifida, the mildest forms of which require no surgery. This particular case is myelomeningocele, one of the most severe types. The spinal cord is right there, exposed in this little sac on the baby's back.

The plan is to close the hole. Before I do that, I'm going to attempt to rebuild the spinal column. You can't create bone, but you can draft in muscle from elsewhere as well as skin.

My job title is 'paediatric neurosurgeon'. Most people would translate this as 'baby brain surgeon', but where babies are concerned the spinal cord is part and parcel of my work. After all, the brain and spinal cord develop from the same line of cells, with one end ballooning up to form the brain and the other literally shrinking away to form the end of the spinal cord. All the relevant developmental steps for spinal cord development within the foetus have been made by day twenty-one of the pregnancy, before the mother even knows there is a baby inside her.

I use my operating loupes when I do these operations. I can see the infinitesimally small and partially opened coverings of the spinal cord, where the bone, muscle and skin of the back used to be. It looks like gossamer. Using a very fine pair of forceps and some really small scissors, I separate off the spinal cord tissue from the coverings and then from the muscle. The hole running down the centre of the cord comes from the ventricle in the brain. The brain fluid should course down and beyond. I basically need to create a new round section of spinal cord. With care I can make out the nerve patterns and find where the central canal should have been. I bring those nerves over, hold them in place and stitch them up. Think of it as like making a swiss roll, but with spinal cord instead of sponge. And then I make another swiss roll around the cord roll, using the gossamer tissue layer, ensuring I don't damage the super-soft neurological tissue.

Next, we find the muscle on the sides – over the pelvis – the defect is almost always in the lower midline area of the back, just above the buttock cleft. My plastic surgeon colleague is well used to working on these areas, so he spends an hour freeing up these muscles and mobilizing them, attached to their blood supply, to allow them to move over the centre where the cord is. He then closes these over, which just leaves the skin.

Babies have soft, stretchy skin. They're like tiny super-cute old men. That's the good news. The bad news is that it's like that for a reason. They are abdominal breathers and they don't tend to use their chests like adults. That's why you see their little tummies pulsating up and down. If you need to pull the skin quite tight around from the front to the back, then with movement and breathing, the wound will be put under tension, and is likely to tear open at the back. The ideal situation is to have the skin nice and lax. Hence the plastic surgeon standing next to me. I can see that we're going to need more than I can stretch from the nearby region.

We take skin from the back, the shoulders, the buttocks – anywhere nearby – to get the newly closed spinal cord area covered. It requires an excellent knowledge of the blood supply of any given part of the skin to ensure that the oxygen keeps flowing to all of it, even as the plastic surgeon cuts it up into a complex latticework to cover the whole area.

It's a methodical procedure, a series of steps that must be taken in sequence. The damage, one has to admit, has already been done, from the perspective that we cannot regain the function of the spinal cord which never developed. But we need to avoid further problems. Some can happen immediately after the operation – infection, leakage of spinal fluid and potential meningitis, wound breakdown, which can lead to the whole area literally falling open again.

Some of these can arise many years in the future. If there is poor coverage, patients can have a lot of pain from the area. Even worse, if they use a wheelchair most of the time, they may end up with pressure sores and possible breakdown of the skin on their back. There may be no recovering from that, as most of the sources of the grafts have been used up in the initial operation. People can literally die from the complications of spina bifida, and from nothing to do with the spinal cord at all.

* * ✦ * *

There is no universally accepted 'cause' for spina bifida. There is some evidence to suggest that a deficiency of folic acid during the early stages of pregnancy can be a trigger. There is also good reason to believe it follows a genetic line. Because we can't emphatically name a cause, parents often blame themselves. Once the stress of the operation was over for the baby, the parents in this case didn't blame themselves. They blamed each other.

'I told you to stop drinking.'

'And I told you to stop smoking.'

'It's your fault. Your whole family's built wrong.'

'What are you talking about?'

'Look at your uncle. You can't tell me he's right in the head.'

'Don't you dare talk about my family.'

And so it goes. We spend some significant amount of time assuaging guilt and recriminations in our job – it's important to try to keep families from needlessly tearing themselves apart in the aftermath of what can often be devastating news.

For parents who, unlike this pair, do adhere to their appointed prenatal scan schedule, there may not be such a shock on delivery day. In a standard case, the sonographer flags the possibility of spina bifida in the foetus at the twenty-week stage, which starts a ripple effect up the chain. Sooner rather than later, I may be called in to discuss the family's options. And by 'options' I mean the worst, most basic kind. I talk to them about the condition, what it means for the child. We discuss treatment plans, and chances for an independent life for the child. This is what parents need to know. But all this feeds into the final decision that they need to make now – keep the baby or don't. Proceed with the birth or go for termination. In a very literal sense, Life or Death. Which do you choose? Left to my own devices, I could wallow in the hell that is explaining that choice. Having that talk with expectant parents is heartbreaking, watching their faces as the brutal reality kicks in. But I need to remember that whatever anguish I'm feeling is nothing – nada – zero – *zilch* – compared to the turmoil I'm about to inflict on two unsuspecting people.

· · ✦ · ·

The couple in front of me are pretty regular. Young, married, first-time parents-to-be. They've just received the hammer blow that their twenty-week miracle has spina bifida. Like a lot of people, they've heard of it, but only vaguely. Like a disease from the history books, typhoid or polio, it's something they're aware of but have never come across. Certainly something they never, ever anticipated when they embarked down the path of starting a family.

I've studied the scans en route. It's a fairly typical case. To me, that is. To the parents it's a once-in-a-lifetime horror show. At these most traumatic of times tears are to be expected. To be encouraged, even, if only to allow parents to accept how big a deal these conditions are.

I cry a lot. Not in front of my patients, but sometimes when I'm alone in my office or on the sofa at home, mulling over what I've seen that day. Mind you, I cry when I watch most Disney films – I haven't yet got through the bit in *The Lion King* when Mufasa dies without tears, so perhaps I would be counted on the 'blubby' end of the population. What I'm saying is, it's a perfectly natural physical and emotional response to terrible news.

Yet the second I walk into a room, I see people desperately trying to stop weeping or pretending the terrible thing never happened in the first place. It's as if they feel ashamed of showing their feelings in front of doctors. Like we're too important or too precious to be bothered by their petty human trifles. Perhaps I'm reading too much into it. Or possibly that's their wider experience. Maybe that's how some medical people want them to be. But it's not how I am. 'Take your time,' I say. 'You've had a shock. We can talk when you're ready.'

I never pull punches with patients, I won't lie to them, I won't sugar-coat the truth. I will, however, go out of my way to deliver it with the softest of velvet gloves at precisely the optimal time. When I sense that the young couple are ready, I start nudging them towards considering their future reality.

'This is what we know of spina bifida,' I begin, and I give them a brief description of the general problem. 'Some babies have more difficulties than others. I'm afraid yours is towards the serious end.'

The 'Can you fix it?' question comes up early. I'm as prepared as I can be. I've delivered the same speech hundreds of times. I could deliver it a thousand times more and it would still pain me the same.

'No, I'm sorry,' I reply. 'I wish I could. The best I can do is stem the pain, minimize the damage that's already there and give your baby the best possible chance at a life worth living.'

Some parents sit there, stunned, silent. Waiting for me to take the lead. Others unleash a barrage of questions to which they don't always want answers. There's no right or wrong way to react. It's two sides of the same emotion: shock. Two reactions to the same impossible situation that they weren't in when they left home that morning.

From what I can see on the scans, I have a good idea of the severity of their baby's condition and can predict, with some accuracy, what the child's life would entail outside of the womb. I give the parents a few moments to process my earlier reply and steady their nerves before sharing the next stage of information. There's no point speaking while they're still in shock. They won't process the words. They won't understand the gravitas. And I really need them to. We're talking about the biggest decision they'll ever have to make in their lives.

We've almost reached the end of the day and I have nowhere to go other than home to my family. My wife and the kids will soon be sitting down to eat, going over the business of their respective days.

The usual chaotic, noisy, glorious mess. They won't be happy that I'm not there, but they're used to it. Used to Daddy running in late, starving, scrabbling around for wherever my dinner is being kept warm – it's always there for me – or my attempts to do a late 'catch-up' of their day while they're trying to relax in bed, or just seeing me the next morning. I hate missing out on any second of their lives. But I know how lucky I am. The alternative is sitting right in front of me.

The parents are now calm, receptive and ready for the next stage. So I begin.

I tell them how their baby might have little or no bladder or bowel function, and that he or she probably won't be able to walk unaided. Sexual function will be limited. Breathing could be difficult. And, worst of all, judging from the inflated size of the brain, quite major developmental problems will almost certainly ensue.

I'm all about the facts. I want the parents to know as much as I do about this particular, unique, special little foetus. I don't want to be overtly negative. When you consider it, a baby doesn't actually *need* bladder and bowel function. None of them have it when they're born. A child doesn't *need* to be able to walk. An adult doesn't *require* sexual function. Most of these problems may seem inconsequential when they're born. When they're two and they're not able to walk, it becomes a bit of a problem, but you can be carried about until you're five or six. When you're sixteen and can't walk? Even then there's a possible workaround, as you can get a wheelchair, you can get a low rider bus, you can physically circumvent almost everything. Psychologically, though, it can be really tough. Some children don't give two hoots and just get on with everything – no issues are too much. But others have a very different reaction.

To be mentally acute and trapped in a dysfunctional body can sometimes break the strongest personalities, especially in teenagers. I've seen it. You look around, see your peers running, dancing, even falling over – you dream of doing any of it. It gets to you.

Everywhere you look there are the constant reminders that 'you're not right' and that 'you need help'. These aren't my words – they are what children actually say to me in clinic. Perversely, if the brain problems are as severe as I predict, and they do significantly delay mental development, the psychological impact of being 'different' is likely not to be as punishing, if it even registers at all.

'Whoopee,' I imagine the parents sarcastically telling me. 'That's such good news, Doctor. You're telling us our baby won't have the mental capacity to even understand how disabled they are ...'

I'm walking a fine line. I only speak of probabilities, not absolutes. Doctors have been wrong before. Miracles have happened.

After ten minutes during which the parents have just sat there mutely, I pause and invite questions. To my mind I've told them everything I can. They're forewarned and forearmed about what's likely to come. They doublecheck one or two things. Ask me to repeat this or that. When I'm satisfied that they're on the same page, I step it up. 'Okay,' I say, 'the choice is up to you.'

And what a choice. I'm not saying, 'Would you like me to improve Baby's leg function or bladder control?' I'm not asking, 'Should we fix this or that?' It's much more primeval. More primitive. The question no parent ever wants to consider: *Would you still like to proceed with your pregnancy?*

I don't say this directly. Not without being asked. Most parents will seek my opinion eventually. They tend to ask two things. The first is: 'What would you do?'

It's such an explosive question. I'm not particularly religious. I'd describe myself as a lapsed Hindu/agnostic. I understand faith in others and I also understand that innate burning fire that drives most – not all – of us to procreate and bring new life into the world. But professionally speaking, my answers focus on two issues that concern the child's welfare: will your child's life be one of an unfair amount of pain and will they have a quality of life that is acceptable to the family and ultimately to them? And I'd also put this question to the parents: *will you be able to cope?*

I'm there to counsel, to advise, to paint a picture of the future. I can't give spiritual direction. But, as a doctor, I can try to describe what life going forward will be like. For the family and, most importantly, for the baby.

Raising a severely disabled child is not for the faint-hearted. I've seen otherwise strong, healthy units destroyed by the addition of a child with special needs. But I've also seen very disabled children having a fantastic quality of life and giving their families unending amounts of joy and happiness. I've seen both outcomes and I can't predict either. The best I can do is present some questions that parents might want to consider.

How able is your family to spend as much time as may be necessary with the new arrival? This could be at the expense of their siblings, of course, or it may turn the siblings into carers – for better or worse. Is the enjoyment that a brother or sister may get from helping look after the baby 'worth' the very rapid growing up they might have to do?

Will your finances affect how much time and care and – harsh as it sounds – attention you can afford to spend on your newborn? Will you hire somebody to be with them or will one of you take a career break to attend to his or her very specific needs? Even if you can afford it financially, will you grow to resent it?

It's a strangely unquantifiable question, but basically, will this family be able to cope with this difficult situation?

I don't know. They don't know. But they are the ones who will have to decide. All I can offer is this: 'Please be honest with yourselves and each other. Now is the time to make hard decisions. Very soon it will be too late.'

The issue in which I am more confident of taking sides concerns the baby's well-being. If I know that it may struggle to breathe unaided, that it will probably require numerous surgical treatments within a short amount of time, that it may not enjoy many moments of peace, then I will say so. As a healthcare professional I can't tell them what to do, but I can tell them what to expect.

The difference is when they ask me what I personally would do. What would Jay the dad do in their shoes? Many of my colleagues avoid this question – and that is probably the right thing to do. But sometimes, the parents REALLY want to know. I am not in their shoes. How do we know how we may react in these situations? Often it is impossible. Of course, I have had three children with my wife, and each of them had an ultrasound scan. We had discussed what we would do if there were problems found with each of them, and we didn't agree with each other.

Sometimes I say, 'Okay, totally without prejudice, just me speaking from the heart, on purely personal grounds, I would not go ahead with this pregnancy. I believe that your baby will have such brain injuries that they will have little or no quality of life. They will also probably undergo more suffering than anyone deserves.'

Other times I say, 'Yes, I would continue if this was mine. Your baby will have problems. They will have a different life to what was wanted or expected. But different is not the same as worse. It's just different. Many people have no disabilities, either physically or developmentally, and basically waste their lives doing nothing useful. Many of my patients, with the sort of problems your baby will probably have, enjoy great lives – and are happy and productive members of society. They have a worthwhile *quality of life*.

'*That* is what I would do.'

The second question I'm asked is much more welcome. 'Can we think about it?'

I'm always pleased when parents want to take the time. It shows consideration. These things shouldn't be rushed. That being said, we do need the decision sooner rather than later. With a termination on the table, facts will only get you so far. What mothers don't want to do is to go from an insensate pregnancy to feeling the baby move. You can talk about all the doomsday science in the world, but that counts for nothing compared to the bond of a mother experiencing that kick or hiccough or stretch for the first time.

Sometimes, people take a day or a weekend. In this case, the family just want a bit of time away from me. They get up to return to the waiting room, But I won't hear of it.

'Stay where you are. Take your time. Relax.' I collect my scans and notes and head back to my own office across campus. 'You have my number. Call me when you're ready.' I say to the specialist midwives who play such a vital part in this care pathway.

I'm barely back at my desk when my mobile rings. They've decided. Or have they? I walk back over.

Their minds are in turmoil, spinning. They both start speaking at once, talking over each other. I let them run on, then calm them down and nod at Mum to go again.

'I worry what people will say if we terminate a baby just because he's a bit poorly. We'll just look selfish.'

Dad adds, 'I worry about bringing a baby into the world that we think is going to be in pain.'

It's two sides of the same coin. A coin I'd prefer them to ignore.

'I know it feels like the eyes of the world are on you, but they're not. It's just you and me in this room. No one's judging you. No one knows exactly what you're going through. It doesn't matter if ninety-nine other people have chosen option A; if you want to choose B, then that's the right choice for you. It is your decision alone to make.'

It's a minefield. A moral and emotional booby trap lining every direction. But I can see in their eyes they have reached a conclusion.

'We've decided not to go ahead,' Mum says.

'You're sure?' I ask.

'It's the right thing.'

I nod. I smile. I try to be positive at this devastating time. From a medical point of view, they've made the decision. The obstetric team will arrange to perform the procedure within twenty-four hours. My time with this family is over. But they will have to live with their decision forever.

＊　＊　◆　＊　＊

Every family is different. Some respond to the bombshell of spina bifida as though a gunman has already taken out their loved ones. Others are more stoic. Some seem almost upbeat. I treat them all the same, offer the same guidance. I'm like a judge. I can't decide the outcome, but I can direct the jury. But sometimes families make decisions that I can't comprehend.

Another young couple were passed my way. Hard-working, good jobs, big prospects. On paper they had decent parent potential. The spina bifida alarm had been sounded as standard. The obstetrician had done his thing, I'd been called over and, as empathetically as possible, had unfurled their future offspring's health chances. They immediately decided to terminate.

In other circumstances I might have admired their clarity of vision. Except in this case, the prognosis wasn't that terrible. Of the levels of severity, this one was as low as I'd seen it. The baby would probably walk, with help. The issues would be likely restricted to the ankles, and maybe some problems with bladder function. The child would almost certainly be able to attend regular school.

In short: would it be perfect? I had to say, 'No, probably not.' Not by the accepted understanding of physical development, but it would be pretty close.

'Then we would like to terminate.'

'Are you sure? There wouldn't be that much …' I'm about to launch into my spiel about quality of life and how their baby would, by all indications, have a good one.

'We're sure. We'd like to terminate the pregnancy.'

I see so much pain in my profession. So many parents anguishing over whether they'd done something wrong. So many babies afflicted by the most terrible of ailments that I find myself wondering whether death might be a blessing. What I see most consistently are parents fighting to secure any chance of a life with their baby.

So, when I'm faced with a scenario where a foetus is being terminated, despite being likely to have had what I would consider a different, but good quality of life, I sometimes struggle. But, as ever, all I can do is lay out the facts. They have to make the decision – it is not up to me. And in this case, a decision has been made with considerable conviction. Who am I to judge?

CHAPTER SIXTEEN

YOU'RE ONE OF THOSE

It wasn't so long ago that spina bifida seemed a much more common diagnosis. Growing up in Liverpool, then London, there were permanent collection tins in shopping centres, adverts offering practical support, regular mentions on current affairs programmes. So what changed?

We all still start life as a ball of cells. We then become a flat plate. We develop a head, a back, a bottom, legs and feet. The skin and the spinal cord come from the same cells. Usually they grow together as fully as expected. But sometimes they don't.

So far, so spina bifida. The only difference is that now we catch it earlier, for which we have advancements in scanning technology to thank. However, an early diagnosis is just part of the story. It's one thing being able to identify with some clarity a potentially life-changing developmental issue, but another to deal with it. It feels like the *really* big change in the management of spina bifida is access to, and deciding whether to have, a procedure for termination.

All the technology in the world is no match for a shift in norms of morality. A modern sonographer can isolate spina bifida with unerring accuracy. But if you live in a culture that's opposed to abortion, what is the point?

* * ◆ * *

The couple I'm about to meet are taking my visit as a courtesy. They've had their twenty-week scan, again as a nod to convention. If ever there were a case of going through the motions, this is it. They didn't want to know the gender of their baby and they certainly weren't concerned with its health. They were pregnant. They were grateful. They were standing on the verge of progressing from being a couple to becoming a family. And nothing was going to prevent it. Not even the prospect of having a child with a severe physical and mental disability.

The obstetrician and I look at the images on the ultrasound machine while he does a new, up-to-date scan. We do this so I can ask questions and he can show me answers, as much as the position of the baby will let him. As far as I can tell, their baby will register at the more severe end of the condition's scale. A large degree of high function will be absent from the second that he or she emerges from the safety of the uterus' cocoon. We'll be lucky if he or she gets to breathe unaided for a single day.

We finish up, and ask them to wait in a counselling room. Then the obstetrician and I talk about the case in private.

'They've really made up their minds,' he says. 'Termination isn't on the table.'

'So they're really determined to go ahead?'

'One hundred per cent,' he replies.

And now for the million-dollar question. 'Religious?'

'What do you think?'

Another redundant question. 'Okay,' I say, 'let's go and see them.'

* * ◆ * *

There are so many variables in medicine. Advances in technology or research can turn an entire field of expertise on its head overnight. It's an effort to keep up. Yet some things never change. All the evidence in the world can be no match for a single person's religious beliefs.

I can never give promises just as I don't touch predictions. I deal in likelihood and best- or worst-case scenario. I follow the evidence and interpret it as best I can. And yet sometimes that prognosis goes out the window, along with my twenty years' experience and more than a decade's worth of training. It can sometimes all count for naught in the eyes of religious or cultural opinion. And it doesn't even matter which. They all appear equally emphatic: babies *must* be born.

* * ✦ * *

I'm surprised to see the family crying. And relieved. The whole stoicism in the face of adversity thing can be unnerving. *Maybe this is not going to be so predetermined after all?*

It's wishful thinking at best. A commitment to God doesn't negate human emotion. I make a note to chastise myself later for my assumptions. It doesn't take long to discern that they are both torn. The Almighty might have the last word, but it doesn't mean they agree with Him. Not entirely, anyway.

'Your scans,' I begin.

'We only did it to be prepared,' Dad interrupts. 'It makes no difference.'

'You're not worried?'

'Of course we're worried. We're besides ourselves. But there is no choice. The baby is coming. We have to be ready. God wills it.'

It's impressive the strength of people's faith in the face of what I think is really, really amazingly bad news. They are upset, they're distraught, but they still take the positives: 'Well, we've got our baby and we're going to love our baby because this is what God has decided.'

I have my script. I trot out the facts, the stats, the evidence, the previous cases that have begun this way and ended well sometimes, badly mostly. I'm giving it the realistic sell. Not quite the big push, but there is a really severe level of problems in this baby. I want them to have a realistic view of what their life, and that of their child, will be like. Yet all the while knowing that I'm shouting into the wind.

I am happy for the family to take all the information we can give them and make either decision. But I feel somewhat frustrated that the facts are irrelevant. Why is that, I often ask myself? Why does it matter to me *why* they make their decision? They have made it – I need to accept it and move along. But, rightly or wrongly, I feel myself trying to make the discussion stay relevant.

'Thank you for seeing us,' Dad says. 'I know you're a very busy man.'

I get the sense he is closing things down.

'I appreciate your efforts and we'll be very happy to have you treat our baby when he or she arrives.'

I *am* being closed down. It's an odd feeling. I'm used to running my own meetings. But then I'm used to being the higher power in the room. Not today. I feel like I'm back in my student days with an overbearing consultant overruling my every decision. Except I could see the consultants. The entity sharing my office now is rather less tangible.

* * ✦ * *

'What do you think?' the obstetrician says, the second I emerge.

'Not sure, if I'm honest.'

'But?'

'But any baby born into a family that really, really wants to give it a great home can't be argued with. How many kids do I send home knowing that they're not going to get half as much love as this baby will?'

We share a moment. Then one of us makes a joke at the other's expense and we go back to our jobs, if not our lives.

Providing healthcare alongside the provisions of faith isn't ever straightforward. Contrary to tabloid belief, overtly religious people don't go around announcing it at every opportunity. Sometimes we're deep into a meeting before I get an inkling of what's driving their narrative. And when I do it's, 'Oh, okay, this is where we are.'

But that's just my personal opinion. It is irrelevant to this set of parents. The family went on to have the baby, and, despite a huge catalogue of problems, operations, hospital visits and stays, I have very rarely seen a child loved so dearly and given such a chance at enjoying life.

· · ◆ · ·

My wife fell pregnant with our first child in 2007. My obstetrician colleague was our go-to guy. Why work with the best if you can't exploit it?

After one such occasion, I walked my wife to the car park before strolling back to my office. By the time I got there, the phone was ringing. It was the obstetrician.

'For God's sake, what did you forget to tell us?' I asked.

'Why does everything have to be about you?' he laughed. 'No. This is different. We've got a case in I think you should see.'

'Okay, I'm on my way.'

The majority of faces that pass through our joint care are youngish; twenties to late thirties. Every so often you meet someone closer to your own age. But that doesn't mean you have any more in common.

The couple I was due to greet were mid-forties, my age essentially, and so, *so* desperate to have a baby. The years had not been kind. Miscarriage had followed miscarriage. They were at their wits' end and expecting the worst when suddenly this latest pregnancy hit the twenty-week mark. It was the furthest they'd ever got. They came rushing in for their scans. They couldn't believe it was happening. They were going to have a baby. And they wanted to see it on the monitors with their own wide, disbelieving eyes.

Unfortunately for them, the scans aren't designed to show what you deserve. They show what you have. And what this couple had was the prospect of life with a severely disabled child. I'd like to say that it was just one of those things, a roll of the dice and it could happen to anyone. That's what your neighbour or your best friend would say to make you feel better. As a neurosurgeon, a man of the disinfected cloth, I held a different view, as harsh as it seemed.

Looking at the couple's charts I saw a myriad of lost attempts. So many pregnancies, so many miscarriages, so much heartache, but no discernible cause. Miscarriages do occur for random reasons, but multiple occasions can suggest a deep-lying problem. Maybe there's a genetic thing going on. Perhaps it's a fatal outcome of the chromosome mix of Mum and Dad. Hell, maybe it's the wrong star signs combining – at this stage nobody knows for sure. All we can go on is the proportion of failures compared to successful pregnancies. And this one did, initially, appear successful. Until the sonographer handed in her homework.

Walking back to see the same obstetrician with whom I'd literally just had my own appointment was a struggle, I'll be honest. Barely twenty minutes ago we'd been talking about my own prospective bonny, healthy, lung-bustingly *normal* baby. Now here I was, alongside the same man, about to counsel two innocent victims of genetic fate. Talk about mixed emotions. I was still buzzing with my own family news until the second he handed over the scans. Then I was on autopilot. I felt all trace of my wife and the baby fade. Jay the dad no longer existed. Jay the neurosurgeon was in the room.

The parents-to-be were perfectly lovely and clearly in love. For obvious reasons I found myself opening up about my own situation. 'Listen, you know what, my wife is pregnant right now. We had our own scans this morning. I know exactly the huge elation you've been feeling up until now and I can only imagine the huge sword that is being passed through you at the idea of having to come and see me. But we've got to get through this, we need to talk about it and then you need to make a plan.'

'A plan?' Dad said. 'Don't we just come back in twenty weeks' time?'

Oh, I realized, *you're one of those.*

* * ◆ * *

I'm so used to being asked my opinion that it can come as a shock when it's not required. If you ask Jay the physician for his views on your situation, he'll tell you facts and conclude, 'But the decision is yours.' If you ask Jay the man – the father – what he would do, he'll say, 'I'd go ahead with the birth' or 'I'd terminate in the interests of the baby's health.' I can't not, as a living, breathing person, have an opinion. I can't not put myself in every single parent's shoes. Though I'd rather not, as it's a horrible place to be.

To decide not to consult an expert at all is a bit like being lost in a desert and having a map but choosing not to use it. If you believe that God will lead you to safety quicker than any science, then why would you ask science?

I get it, I do. At least I think I do. I think sometimes I am religious, but just really *pissed off* at what God is letting happen in the world and to my patients. At other times, I decide I don't believe at all. Is that petulance because God isn't doing what I expect him/her to do? Who knows? And anyway, I need to leave that at the door. Like Dr McCoy almost said in *Star Trek*, 'Dammit Jim, I'm a doctor, not a Hindu'. That would have been an awesome episode, by the way.

Even though on a census they might identify as Christian, most of the Caucasian native population of Britain – for want of a better overall description – are not particularly religious. They arrive, I advise, I guide and they base their decisions on my input. They're all very grateful that these options are there.

But not so much the devout. Not the extremely religious of any faith. In my experience, they tend to put their religious views above even their personal views. I can see a lot of them are very torn by the decisions that they make. Their instincts as parents – as humans – are screaming one thing, but their training, their upbringing, their allegiance and their fealty to the flock dictates another path. 'This is what God wants.'

I'm just a man in an invisible white coat. I can't argue with that.

I can see the parents in front of me are more torn than they are letting on. In a strange way, so am I. Up until the moment of their child's birth, these two mature adults are my patients. The second we have delivery, their concerns will radically reduce on my radar. I'll be all about the baby. That is, if we get that far.

I still haven't worked out if a termination will be decided here. I have a few more probabilities and possibilities I need to get through to them before they make up their minds.

'To be clear,' I say, 'your baby, should you go full term, is never going to enjoy a life as you and I experience it. Your child is, as close as certainty allows, probably going to need multiple operations. They may be dependent on a ventilator for the rest of their life. And by life I mean "short life". The expectancy for a patient with so severe a condition is probably measured in months or single years.'

The pair are nodding. I honestly think I might be making headway. A few more stats and perhaps I can stop and get their opinion.

'We understand the difficulties,' Dad says. 'Yes, our baby's life might be short. But that short life is important to us.'

'Okay,' I reply. 'If that's your decision, then I shall support your choice.'

I'd like to say my prognosis was wayward, that the baby's afflictions weren't half as severe as I'd predicted. But I can't. He arrived eighteen weeks later in dire need of surgical intervention. The only consolation was that we were forewarned. Everything was set up. From birth to the first ventilator took minutes not days.

On top of everything else, the baby had severe chromosomal anomalies, a really damaged brain and no end of problems. In between every visit to theatre he was put on a ventilator.

Every procedure went like clockwork. We achieved the maximum I hoped we could. But it was never enough. We were always fighting a rising tide. Trying to build a sandcastle as the waves encroached further up the beach.

After the first operation I spoke to the parents. 'Listen,' I said, 'it's looking really bad here. We need to think about how far you want to go.'

They squeezed each other's hands and Mum replied, 'We want you to continue to go all the way. If God wants it to, this will work out.'

'Okay.'

It was the same curt conversation following the second procedure and the third. Before I was due to operate for a fourth time I said, 'I have to be honest. Your child is not going to get better from this intervention. Your child will eventually die. I estimate within weeks, but it's possible it may take months. This is no way for him to live.'

To which Dad responded, 'Can you be absolutely sure? Can you give us an absolute guarantee that this child cannot survive at all?'

And, you know what? I couldn't. Sometimes being 99.9 per cent sure just isn't enough. 'No,' I said, 'I'd be really surprised if it happened, but I can't give that cast-iron guarantee.'

He turned to his wife. They smiled at each other and kissed. Then, looking back at me, he replied, 'Well, in that case, it's not up to you. It's up to God to decide. So please, do your job, keep going. Do everything you can.'

I shrugged. Not because I didn't care, but I didn't see any point arguing with them. At the end of the day I am a servant to the patient rather than the parents, and if we really wanted to, we could make this a legal fight. But I didn't wish to do that. This poor family were struggling and needed support. Sure, they had it from God, but that's also partly our role. But I needed to ensure we were always keeping my little patient's needs at the top.

'I'm not sure you understand the severity of your son's condition. It is my professional opinion that if your child stops breathing, we shouldn't put him back on the breathing machine again. If we do, he's probably going to be there for life.'

'Sir, you possess wonderful abilities and skills because God has given them to you. Please show your gratitude by continuing His will.'

For two months the baby never left the hospital. Never went home. Never experienced life without being plugged into one machine or other. The parents were regular visitors. One or both was present for a few hours every permitted session although, as the weeks became months, those visits grew shorter and shorter. The ward nurses, on the other hand, were there permanently. They had to be. They tended the boy, cared for him, cleaned and fed him. Like they do for all patients. It can be hugely distressing for these deeply caring women and men to look after the same child for too long. Attachments are great, but if the outcome is bad they can be a weapon turned. The nurses tend to rotate around patients to avoid this, but if you are on there long enough, you will end up being the object of affection of all the nurses. I watched, on day seventy, as they began their morning procedures. Strolling over, I asked, 'How's he doing?'

'He's not happy,' one of them replied. 'Watch the monitor as I clean him.'

I did. I saw how his heart rate spiked when the damp cotton-wool ball touched his tiny body. You'd expect some kind of reaction, but this was higher, more akin to distress.

'Everything hurts,' she said. 'It's not right.'

I couldn't agree more. I just needed two other people to do the same. Or rather, I just had to persuade one of them ...

* * ◆ * *

It's very rare that two adults, two parents, agree 100 per cent on every topic. Dinners, sugar, screen time, bedtime, swearing, chores – you name it, there's wriggle room between parents on every topic. I am betting the farm that this more serious topic would be even more divisive.

'I'll speak to them again,' I promised one of the nurses. 'When do you expect Mum in?'

'Well, she was here for twenty minutes yesterday around lunchtime. I suppose she'll do the same today.'

I realized the nurse was having a dig at the parents, but in an odd way I took it as 'good' news. The fact that Mum and Dad were winding down their visits, downgrading them if you like, told me that on some subconscious level they were resigned to losing. Losing the fight with the disease, losing the son they had yet to hold. It's surprisingly common for parents in pain to drift away. It's like throwing up a wall between them and their pain. If they can't see the baby, they can't be hurt.

'Bleep me immediately when the mum arrives,' I asked the nurse. 'I need to have a chat.'

It was closer to 3 o'clock in the afternoon when I got word she was in the house. I ran down to the special-care baby unit, and accidentally-on-purpose bumped into her.

'Any change?' she asked, forlornly.

'No,' I replied, 'but I think you already knew that.'

She sighs.

'Look,' I said, 'I know you believe that a greater power deigns this to be so. And I respect that, I do. But I have to say, you are not my patient. My loyalty – my moral and legal loyalty – is with that tiny baby attached to the breathing machine in the incubator. And I am telling you that subjecting him to any more treatments is not going to get him better.'

'But …' she began, then faltered.

I continued. 'I think our choices are hurting him. Causing

him pain he need not suffer. There is no medical justification for continuing treatment for your baby. He's not getting better, he will never get better and every day that he draws assisted breath is another day of hurt and distress for him. Now, as a surgeon, as doctors, we do cause pain to babies all the time, but that is part of a treatment that we think will get them better. That isn't what is happening here. Please, speak with your husband.'

· · ◆ · ·

Eventually, the dad came round. We agreed that the child had no real hope of survival. We just stopped artificially forcing him to stay alive. We focused our work on ensuring the baby would be comfortable and pain free. The end was natural and peaceful. Both parents were in shock. They'd put their faith in the Lord showing their son the way. Perhaps, after all, it had been a test. I'm inclined to think that's how they interpreted it.

I have to be honest. This was the outcome I thought was needed. Did it give me any satisfaction to prove the parents wrong? No. Zero. My feelings are with my patient, the little mite who struggled in vain to survive against remarkable odds. If I couldn't help him, I just wanted to comfort him. Finally, I'd done that.

I'm confident, following conversations with both parents, that no one could argue we'd not done our best. Put a gun to my head and we could have kept that baby alive for weeks more. But that would not have been in the baby's interests. Or, ultimately, those of his family. I know we did what was right for that child. And I'm comfortable with that.

Dad eventually came to that conclusion, too. When the tears dried up, he shook my hand and thanked me for my efforts and for doing my best for his son. As much as I disagreed with his original logic, I was proud at that moment. For weeks we'd been at ideological loggerheads. At last we were on the same page. Each of us had only ever had his baby's best interests at heart, we could all see that now.

Or, as the obstetrician put it, 'You got him to admit that you were the only higher power?'

'I did nothing of the sort,' I replied. 'I'm just grateful he didn't accuse me of murdering his baby.'

Because, trust me, that goes on as well …

CHAPTER SEVENTEEN

YOU'RE TRYING TO MURDER OUR BABY!

It's human nature to try to establish order from chaos. To posture as though you're in control of your surroundings. It's a point of principle that my department operates with no real waiting lists. If you need to be seen, you will be seen. Not in six months, not in six weeks, but today or tomorrow. I won't necessarily be there, but one of my team will be. Our business tends not to be the kind that fits well with waiting.

So much of our work is about planning. But some things you cannot anticipate. Like a ten-year-old boy running out into traffic. When the alarm rings we go running. Drop everything, forget everything, get your arse over to A&E or PICU – the Paediatric Intensive Care Unit. He was a local kid, so was naturally brought into our A&E. The second they twigged it was brain trauma, our number was called.

The first responders had the full card. 'Ten-year-old male, road traffic accident, suspected serious head injury.'

To look at the boy you'd never guess what he'd been through –

what he was *still* going through. There were a few facial abrasions and mild bruising to the scalp, but no more than if he'd come off his bike. We probably all experienced worse as kids.

I performed the light test by shining a small torch in his eyes. The pupils reacted, which indicated brain activity. Always a good sign. It meant there was somebody home. The question was, for how long?

Breathing was clearly a problem. The boy's body was not really making a great deal of respiratory effort. Before we did anything else, he needed to be hooked up to a ventilator.

A CT scan is a fairly rudimentary test, but it does give a ballpark picture. And this boy's picture did not look good. Whatever mild state his face and hands were in, his brain was shot. It looked as though the boy had spent some time in a boxing ring. I could only imagine the degree of impact to have shaken things up so violently. And I wasn't the only one thinking about it.

Giving birth can be such a traumatic experience. Babies are, by definition, so defenceless, so weak, so dependent on grown-ups to fulfil all their needs. For first-time parents it can be a testing time, not knowing what you're doing, whether you're doing it right, whether you're doing it often enough. We all go through it. But at some point, things begin to settle down. You realize you do know what you're doing, you love your baby and everything is going to be all right. And then something like this happens.

Imagine ten years of sweet, contented family life. Reflect on all the milestones you go through, all the laughter and tears and experiences shared between parents and child. See yourself looking back and wondering where all the time went, then looking forward and plotting a lifetime of potential achievement. Think of packing your son's sandwiches in his bag, kissing him on his head and setting him off for school, just like you've done so many times before. Then imagine getting the call to say he's unconscious in hospital. Nothing in this world prepares you for that.

We're transporting the boy from A&E to the PICU when a nurse tells me the news I've been expecting and dreading. 'The parents are here.'

'Okay,' I say. 'Get them comfortable. I'll be out as soon as we're done in here.'

What I don't say is: 'Tell them the bad news.' That's my job. It's not something I enjoy, but I know how to do it. I know I can share terrible news, wreck people's lives on occasion, and later process it in a way that enables me, only a little bit broken, to go home to my own family at night. This nurse might be built the same way. She might be able to distance herself from the personal agony of imparting such devastating information. Or she might find herself permanently scarred by the knowledge that she's broken two people's hearts on a random Tuesday afternoon in May. It's not a risk I intend to take.

He's my patient. It's my responsibility. If there are to be tears and acrimony, I want them directed at me. I'm tall, I've broad shoulders literally and metaphorically, as well as a big belly. I can take it. But first, we have to do what we can to save him.

A massive brain trauma is much like twisting your ankle. You don't really know how severe it is until the next day. I know from the scans that what I'm basically looking at is some really bad brain damage. The fact that the boy's eyes are responding is a good sign. I want to know if they're the extent of his abilities or the beginning. To do that, one of the things I need to monitor is the pressure of his brain against the skull. Conditions like hydrocephalus, bleeding or brain swelling can form at any time. We need to be ready.

To do anything we need to get inside without causing any more damage. Luckily, there's a doorway to Narnia. Amazing as it sounds, given how incredibly intricate the brain is and how easily one can destroy a life with just a millimetre's inaccuracy, there are actually places within that we don't really use. If you look at the face and take a line up from the right pupil and intersect it with a line from the top of the ear, there's the right frontal lobe – a quiet part of the brain that just sits there and doesn't seem to do that much. Perhaps in a few years we'll discover that it's a more important part of the whole structure. But based on what we know today, it's generally just padding or filler, which makes it the perfect location for an intracranial pressure monitor.

The boy is under. The anaesthetic will keep him calm. I barely need ten minutes. While I watch, the junior doctor makes a little nick in the skin in the right frontal region, and then drills a small hole, about the size you would put in your wall when hanging up a small picture. Through that, she feeds in a piezoelectric wire. It's basically a fancy version of the technology you use to light a gas ring on a cooker: press the ignition, an electrical charge passes along the cable and it triggers combustion with the gas emission. In this instance, when the brain compresses around the wire, it causes a current which gets converted into pressure and is measured by our pressure machine in millimetres of mercury (mmHg). A normal reading would be between 5 and 10 mmHg.

A few seconds after the wire goes in, I check the monitor. It shows 16 mmHg, which is borderline high, but not out of control. *Maybe* we'll be okay. But just like twisting an ankle, the real swelling is probably yet to come.

I sigh, pull down my mask and wash my hands. Now for the tricky part. Time to talk to the parents.

There's no right way to deal with stress. Often I meet parents who choose to stand apart, on opposite sides of the room, one facing this way, one facing the other. It's not intentional. They don't mean to put up such a disunited front. They're responding as individuals, as humans, as best they can. Others seem determined to share the same body space. They're so close as to cast a single shadow. And I'm looking at a single shadow now.

I begin by offering my sincerest condolences for their pain. I can't imagine what they're going through as parents. It would be presumptuous even to project. But that doesn't mean I can lie to them.

'I have to be honest,' I begin, 'your son is not in a good way. Our initial tests show his brain has suffered a severe injury. It may well prove to be unsalvageable. As unimaginable as it may seem, I need to prepare you for the worst.'

There's silence. Then Dad says, 'By worst you mean … ?'

I nod. He knows the answer. She knows the answer. But I have to say it. 'We're running tests right now and obviously we're doing everything we can. But, I'm sorry to say, there is a real chance your son will die from this injury.'

They nod. They're quiet. They're huddled together as one. When they cry, it's into each other's shoulders.

. . ✦ . .

Just because the prognosis seemed fatal, it didn't mean we were giving up. Far from it. As expected, within six hours there was a serious change in the cranium. The brain was swelling at a pace that would prove catastrophic if left untreated. I needed a theatre slot *tout de suite*.

The results of a follow-up scan confirm in pictures what the piezoelectric reading said in numbers. The brain is swollen and still growing. The pressure on the skull is nearing breaking point. Everyone in the room knows what needs to happen, but I announce it anyway, in my best surgeon's voice: 'We need to do a decompressive craniectomy on this boy.' In shorthand we sometimes say we are going to 'pop the top'. We will be removing large portions of the skull and opening the dura up to allow the brain space to swell.

The 1980s 'Throwback Thursday' music starts and we begin.

✦

Swelling in the brain causes so much pressure that it starts to restrict the flow of blood. In a healthy body, when the heart pumps it pushes the blood up through the blood vessels and supplies oxygen to the brain. Usually, there is no opposition. With a swelling brain, however, those vessels are essentially being compressed, which leads to hypoxia – a reduction in oxygen supply. This then causes injury to the brain and makes it swell up. It becomes a vicious cycle where the swelling causes less oxygen delivery, which causes more swelling, then reduces oxygen flow, ad infinitum or death … Hence the need to pop the top.

We could say 'lift the hood' or 'open the bonnet' or any of the other terms that car mechanics use. But 'pop the top' does it so succinctly. We need to see the meat of the matter and there's only one way in.

The mere act of cutting away the crown of the skull halves the pressure reading. For the change to be so drastic, the boy's brain must have been so tightly compressed. Within ten minutes, however, the brain is beginning to expand again.

I feed an external ventricular drain into the middle of the brain. The idea is to remove the cerebrospinal fluid. The goal is to give the brain tissue enough space to try to fight back. Everything I do is a step in the right direction. I know that, because the pressure on the brain drops. But only briefly. I close the skin over the angry brain. We sit and watch for a while in theatre. Nothing I do prevents the pressure heading upwards.

I only have so many options. When I've exhausted them all, I find myself staring at this battered and bruised young head. What does it want? What is it fighting for? It's mesmerizing. Like watching a pot on the stove. What should be 1.5 kg of solid brain matter is a malleable ballooning mush. Even if I get it back to normal size, I'm not sure what there is left to save.

Another scan confirmed my fears. The brain was disintegrating. To all intents and purposes it was melting, beginning to wipe itself out. With the pressure under control and the 'top' popped back on, the boy was returned to PICU. While the family went outside to make some calls, I left the child under the watchful eye of the intensive care team. It was barely half an hour before I was summoned back.

Nurses are wonderful people, professional and empathetic. They see things and do things on a daily basis that would mentally scar a 'normal' person for years. Even so, watching two twenty-somethings deal with what was coming out of my patient had me marvelling at their capabilities. One had her hand over where I'd stitched up the boy's head. The other was providing swabs and disposing of dirty ones.

'Is this what I think it is?' asked one, plugging the flow with her fingers.

I grimaced. 'Yeah, I'm afraid so. It's brain.'

I remember being in Glasgow, years ago, and rushing in to find nurses in a similar situation. I was a newbie then, fresh off the boat medically speaking, quite impressionable and easy to shock. I looked on, enthralled as this mature Scottish lady lovingly sponged the emissions from the patient's head. When she saw me watching, she held up her wet tissue and said, 'Well, that's his school memories gone.'

It's dark humour, hideously so, but what else can you do? The nurse then was literally wiping away smears of a patient's brain, just as the young women in front of me, twenty years later, were doing. Imagine squeezing a toothpaste tube and watching the last dregs ooze out. That is what I was witnessing. Brainy 'paste' was seeping inexorably from the holes where the stitches had been put in. It looked like bloody rice pudding. The brain was obviously taking on water and getting soft and mushy as part of the dying process. I really felt for the nurses. No one should have to do that.

Such a terrible sight had to be kept from the parents, so we put a bandage on the boy's head.

* * ◆ * *

Mum and Dad soon returned from phoning their relatives – what a job. I talked them through what had happened, and we decided to wait and see how things would develop. They had not left the hospital once in the thirty-six hours since their son had been admitted. I'd kept them as up to date as I could, briefing them before and after all the various procedures. Some chats were more detailed than others depending on time and knowledge. I pulled my punches, a little bit. They didn't need to know all the gory details. What I didn't do, however, was deviate from the truth of the matter which was, essentially, 'Your boy is not likely to survive.'

As the hours and days went on, they grew more resigned to his fate. Or so I thought.

The time finally came for me to have 'The Conversation'. Again, it's not a job I would ever countenance asking anyone else to endure. The parents had fresh coffees when I found them in the waiting room. I was in my blues, having just emerged from theatre. I brought my PICU consultant colleague with me, as we always try to do this as a team. I had a rough idea of what I was going to say and a rough idea of how they'd respond.

So I began. I recapped all the efforts we'd made to keep their child alive. None of it was fresh news to the parents. At the end I said, 'Despite our best efforts, there is nothing else to be done. It is my suggestion that we let your son die.'

Everyone takes the news in their own way. Generally, I've got to know people well enough to predict how they'll be. This pair, I was confident, would understand and accept their fate, never forgetting the heartbreak. In reality, it was quite the opposite response.

'Why would you stop?' Dad asked. 'He's alive, isn't he? His heart is still beating.'

'Yes, it is, but his brain is not working.'

'But his heart is. That means he's breathing. He's alive.'

I let the conversation move around the dance floor a little, going nowhere, then pointed into the PICU. 'You know that bandage around your son's head? It's there because his brain is so damaged and swollen that it is actually leaking through the incision in his skin. That's a really, *really* bad place to be.'

As fireside chats go, it was like using a sledgehammer to crack a nut, but I was stumped by their reaction so far. And still it didn't work.

'You're our doctors,' Dad said. 'Don't let our son down. Please keep working.'

It was an awful situation. The boy was as good as brain-dead. I hadn't yet conducted a brainstem test to check for brain death, but I was pretty sure of the final result. I tried once again to explain the severity of the situation to the parents.

'If we'd done nothing when your son arrived he would have died. If at any stage since he's been here that we hadn't acted, he would have died. His brain is dying if not dead. He is being breath-assisted by a machine. Apart from minimizing his pain, there is very little we can do.

'As long as he is alive, you have to help him,' Dad replied. 'We want you to. It is the law.'

Yes, I thought, *yes, it is. But the law also has provisions for cases like these.*

There was nothing more to be done. We could replace the bandages, clean the exit wound, supply pain relief and anaesthetics, and make sure the ventilator stayed plugged in. Nothing else was going to change. No new brain was going to evolve. Junior wasn't ever likely to spring back into life.

I left it overnight and approached the family once again the next day. This time I was more emphatic. I had the measure of them now. 'My medical advice to you both is that we disconnect him from the ventilator. He won't breathe for himself, but we will make sure he is not in any pain or distress. We can be in a side room and you can be with him when he passes away.' Or words to that effect.

Honestly, I don't think it would have mattered what I said. The very insinuation that this couple's hard-fought, first-born child would have his life support extinguished drove the dad, in particular, to despair.

'I don't believe this,' he shouted. 'You're trying to murder our baby!'

He squared right up to me. He pushed his chest into mine. Our eyes locked. The saving grace was that mine were about 6 inches higher than his. I towered over him. I was the wrong person to be physically intimidated. I'm big, I can soak it up. Of course, if he'd done the same thing to one of my staff, particularly one of the slighter nurses, it could have been a very different story. In such situations you have to let the parents vent. I knew it was painful. I knew it was an unpleasant truth to face. Even so, I had to say it. 'I'm not trying to murder anyone. To all intents and purposes, your son is already dead.'

* * ◆ * *

The truth of the matter was, very simply, that their son had been as good as killed by the car that hit him. He was currently dying on one of our beds not *because* of our treatment, but *despite* it. We had done everything in the playbook to extend that poor soul's chances.

I decided to give it another couple of hours before I broached the subject with the parents again. As it turned out, I didn't get the chance.

I was back in my office, prepping for another case, when the phone rang. It was reception at the PICU. 'Could you come down please, Jay? There are two people here to see you.'

'Okay,' I said. 'Who are they?'

'I didn't catch the names, but one of them is a police officer.'

* * ✦ * *

It's the quiet ones you have to watch out for. Dad was forty-five, middle class and as average as you could imagine. Obviously well kept, well dressed, well mannered. Nothing about him was pompous or snobby or aggressive. He'd probably never said boo to a goose his entire life. But on this occasion, he was making waves. I'd seen it before. He was Daddy Bear looking out for his cub.

The only thing I'd never seen before was a police officer, investigating ME.

I relayed the events of the previous forty-eight hours. Because he was the victim of a road traffic accident, the police already had the boy's details on file. When I'd finished explaining, the lead guy said, 'Right, okay, so what you're telling us is this boy has a completely unsurvivable injury and you're suggesting that you stop treatment?'

'It's standard procedure,' I said. 'So yes.'

'Well then, you're okay. That's not really a crime. Not even close.'

The policemen were as apologetic as they could be. I got it, I understood. They'd had a visit at the station from a stressed, anxious, terrified father accusing me of heinous behaviour. They had a duty to investigate. Now they had a duty to repair the damage. Up to a point.

'Can you do me a favour and tell the dad that I have no choice but to stop treatment here?'

'Yeah, well, we could,' the officer said, smiling grimly – the sort of smile I only see from coppers, firemen, ambulance techs, nurses and doctors. It's the smile of people who have seen the ass-end of life, who've witnessed what people can do to each other and the terrible circumstances they're forced to endure. 'But maybe that would be better coming from you.'

And with that they were gone. The cowards, I thought, jealously.

Dad took this development as well as could be expected. Which is to say, he buried his head further in the sand. 'I don't care what the police say,' he said. 'I forbid you to terminate my son's life.'

No amount of reasoning was going to work. It was time to bring in the big guns.

· · ✦ · ·

When I'm in theatre, when I have Talking Heads or whoever blasting out, I become detached from the world around me and can imagine I'm all alone. In that moment, I'm exactly where I need to be. If I'm honest, I'm rarely happier.

But there is an outside world and I am actually part of a much larger organization. Too often that organization is just a conduit for excessive paperwork and unnecessary meetings. Occasionally, though, it's a godsend, like when you're seeking to make a patient a ward of court.

I gave my boss the heads-up. Then I spoke to the doctors in the PICU and we filled out the relevant forms. The boy was technically their patient. Between the two departments we had a concrete deposition for court.

Most people have experienced the 'law's delay'. If this were a motion to get a child rescued from neglect, I'd expect it to take a week or two. For this particular case that would not do.

I didn't attend court, but I got the message that we'd been successful. A judge had squeezed the application into his schedule and made the decision. We – the hospital, the doctors – were now the legal guardians of this poor little boy.

I took no pleasure from 'winning' this particular battle. It basically meant we had the authority to cease giving care to a ten-year-old boy. On what planet would that be called a win?

Unlike me, Dad had gone to court. He'd railed at the judge, done everything he could to get the motion denied. The judge commented that he clearly loved his son but, in this instance, the right thing to do wasn't necessarily the instinct of a parent.

It was only late in the day that I got the news that the parents were very religious. A nurse on the PICU ward told me on the phone that they were seeking spiritual guidance. Later that day, a vicar arrived to speak with them.

I had high hopes for the outcome. But they were misplaced. The dad chucked the clergyman out on his ear yelling, 'You're all in it together!'

Okay, I thought, *I tried. But now it's time ...*

Even with the full might of the law on your side, there is no easy way of imposing it. I wasn't dealing with a madman, a psychopath or someone who was out to hurt or maim another. I was in the presence of a dad torn apart by his desire to save his family. Whatever happened, there would be no winners here today. Not him and certainly not his son.

We always invite loved ones to be involved in last contact. They might want to hold their child's hand, to pray or just be present in the room, but perhaps looking the other way. It makes no odds to me. As long as everyone gets the ending they need.

Four days in, Dad was unrecognizable from the man who'd physically threatened me. His shoulders were sagging, his hair unbrushed. He was a broken man. He felt he had let his family down. I could see it in his eyes.

We had not just rushed in once the legal decision was made. We had left it in the background, an unspoken decision about the direction of travel. But this poor man was in probably the worst place anyone could be. About to lose a child. I see it all the time, but it never gets easier. It never stops piercing my attempts to protect myself from my work, like tiny little stab wounds that will no doubt eventually do me in. I am lain bare every time I have the conversation. In fact, I am not ashamed to say that I have wept while correcting this chapter, just remembering this man. Perhaps I am not the best person to do my job, I often think. But then again, where else would I be?

We walked silently over to the PICU. Everyone was made comfortable. Then we disconnected the boy from his ventilator. His oxygen levels dropped. I could see it on the machine. I witnessed him not making any kind of struggle. Shortly afterwards, his heart flickered then stopped completely, joining his brain. He was dead. It was over.

We did our best. All of us. Medical team and family. We all had that little ten-year-old's best interests at heart. We just had different ways of going about it.

CHAPTER EIGHTEEN

IT'S YOUR DECISION

For people of a certain generation, the idea of a consultant doing his ward rounds conjures up the memory of James Robertson Justice from the old *Doctor in the House* film and its many sequels. As Sir Lancelot Spratt, he'd burst through the ward doors, barking orders to the following phalanx of wide-eyed juniors, while the sisters and nurses would swoon at his every word and patients would react like Moses experiencing a visitation from God. Ah, those were the days.

There are still people who bend the knee to anyone in authority, or at least to those wearing a lanyard. White coats, ties, sleeves with cufflinks – all gone. My parents' generation is probably the last that unquestioningly revere every utterance from policemen, teachers, doctors and – at the uppermost of the food chain – the Royal Family. Kids today would rather trust Google than an adult with qualifications and a lifetime's experience. Hell, they'd rather put their faith in Wikipedia. Even politicians have made careers out of poo-pooing 'experts' and the 'establishment'. And that's all going rather well ...

I think the Internet has provided a much-needed shake-up of the status quo, but like everything it can go too far. And, as with many modern innovations, they're fine until they affect you negatively.

Putting your trust in a doctor takes a special kind of faith. You have to believe to your bones that the person advising you not only knows what they're talking about, but also has your best interests at heart. As far as being an expert is concerned, as a doctor you never stop learning – there are papers about new advancements being published all the time. Discussions with peers and keeping abreast of the subject can be a full-time job in itself and it's plausible that the odd new wonder drug or technique could slip under the radar. I do my best. But if a colleague or even a patient can produce some evidence that I'm unaware of, I'll take it on board. Read the paper, do a bit of digging, apply my own expertise. There's no ego here. Or rather, there is an ego, but it would never be the reason that I didn't do something.

As far as having the patient's best interests at heart is concerned, I would be distraught if anyone ever accused me of not putting their child first. Bearing in mind that my wife and I met in Glasgow before I began to specialize, she's seen me progress and grow as a clinician. I can't say she's impressed by the baggage that accompanies it. Twenty years later, according to her, I'm indistinguishable from the job I do. In her opinion, being a paediatric neurosurgeon defines who you are as a person much more than other careers. Most people could switch jobs and remain exactly the same. Not so for my line of work, apparently. She says I am completely 'The Job'. Everything – her, my children, my hobbies, my health – they all fit around the job.

There's no malice intended, and she is proud of the fact that I have so many other 'kids'! However, she also worries about the toll it takes on me – I know that during the frequent debriefs we have, it can sometimes get too much for my little brain to cope with. While hearing all this doesn't necessarily make me feel great as a father or indeed as a husband, it is probably true. But I'd say it's *because* I'm a father that I am as obsessed as I am.

The same thing goes through my mind every time I have a new case. *What if it was one of my own children who needed treatment?*

I would definitely want a doctor who was prepared to drop everything if needed – even if it did mean occasionally letting down his loved ones back home. So that's the guy I try to be.

$$\cdot \quad \cdot \quad \blacklozenge \quad \cdot \quad \cdot$$

Regardless of the personal sacrifices we make, for a parent to trust me to do what I do requires an extraordinary leap of faith. I remember standing outside the operating theatre while my daughter had her tonsils out. I know the surgeon – a great lady, eminent in her field, more than capable of this routine procedure – but even so, handing your child over to someone who is going to take a scalpel, or worse, to her is a test of parenting.

Of course, I have no real way of assessing whether I could do more. My own experience of being the father of a patient is limited. It's one thing giving your precious bundle of joy to someone who says he can fix their broken leg. What must it feel like authorizing me to go to work, knowing I'm going to have to put my fingers in your child's brain?

There's a huge difference between another sort of surgeon saying, 'This is a routine operation. We do ten thousand of them with no problems at all' and me popping the top of your child's skull and admitting, 'This is a major risk operation from which they may not recover or even survive. Consequences abound for personality, language, learning – in fact, everything that makes us human.'

I've seen people have less faith in their own deities than they do in us at that moment, with their child's life on the line. They want us to succeed so desperately that they're prepared to throw their lot in with this person whom they've known for such a short time and give him carte blanche to do anything. Or so it usually goes …

$$\cdot \quad \cdot \quad \blacklozenge \quad \cdot \quad \cdot$$

A young boy came in with a brain tumour. My colleague on duty was perfectly capable of making the diagnosis and leading the surgical response. However, once the MRI results were in, she asked me to come and help her discuss the permutations with the family. She hadn't been a consultant in the department long, and we tend to do some of these lengthy cases as a gruesome twosome. It's always good to have another pair of eyes in theatre.

I was as upfront as ever with the family. 'Your boy has a sizable tumour on the back of his brain. Further specialist scans will show us the extent and we need to check the spinal cord, but it is imperative we begin the process of tackling the tumour immediately.'

'Will you be able to cut it out?' Mum asked.

'We will cut out what we can reach. There may be some parts that are too interwoven with crucial areas. To attempt to attack those could risk further damage.'

'Can you fix him?'

'I have to say, from the evidence of the MRIs it does not look promising just with surgery. We want to remove as much as we safely can, then let's see what's what. Then we can plan the next steps. But I can't promise anything. This is a very dangerous procedure. We will be negotiating with the most sensitive area in the body. There is a small chance your son may not recover from the surgery itself, and may die as a result.'

It's no way to be talking about an eleven-year-old. No way to be speaking to a loving parent. But those were the facts. Sugar-coating them – or lying – would not prepare either parent or child for any future that awaited.

The operation goes as well as can be expected. The music is loud, the stakes are high, the tension in the room is comfortably the right side of manageable. It drives us onwards to be better rather than fearful. We've all been here before, performed the same operation hundreds of times on hundreds of unique brains. We need our wits about us, but I can't see any obvious problems.

Two hours later, we've managed to remove 90-something per cent of the tumour. It's in a pot next to me, vile and selfish. The fact that the human body can generate such a thing to hurt itself is one of life's mysteries. The samples we sent to the pathology were looked at under the microscope. The results have come back almost diagnostic of a particular malignant tumour – something that would be confirmed in a few days. We begin the process of closing the wound. In my head I formulate my report to the mother.

There have been no unforeseen hitches. No hiccoughs of any kind. We went in and achieved what we set out to. If the immediate high-resolution post-op scans come back clear, then perhaps, with radiology and chemotherapy, the boy has a shot at life. But they don't.

After three days, we finally received the pathology and the post-op images with the spinal views. It was terrible news. The tumour had been busy. Secondary malignant growths – 'metastases', as we call them – had spread all down the spine. Everywhere I looked was a new metastasis outcrop.

The conversation I was about to have with Mum was also something I'd done hundreds of times. And, like the brain, they were all unique. I knew what I had to say, but I wouldn't know how I was going to say it until I was face to face with the family. The words had to match the vibe. I couldn't be responsible for adding to their pain any more than I needed to. A little boy had just undergone successful intensive surgery. The expectations for good news were immense.

Mum got the first word in. 'Did you do it? Did you cut it out?'

'Yes,' I replied, 'but …'

'So he's okay?'

'No, please, I have to tell you. While we did pretty well on the tumour, I'm afraid that's just the start of his troubles. It's spread throughout the spinal column. We've found multiple metastases.'

'What does that mean?'

'It means your son is going to need intensive follow-up treatment with chemotherapy and radiotherapy. But this puts him very much on the back foot already.'

I paused. She processed.

'Is there nothing … ?' she said. 'You can't cut out these meta-things?'

Performing life-saving or life-changing operations is the epitome of life as a paediatric neurosurgeon. It's where we really come into our own. Save the life of a child? What greater gift can anyone offer the world?

Yes, it takes training to dance among the brain cells; yes, it takes skill; yes, it takes a lifetime of servitude to the cause. But occasionally it can be the easy way out. The real test of being a good paediatric neurosurgeon is recognizing when operating is not the best option, and being willing and able to share the news, however discomforting it may be. It's about treating the whole family as your patient and not just the unlucky one in the hospital bed.

Let's be blunt. The easy option in most scenarios for surgeons in full-time employment with the NHS is to do another operation. Why not? You're paid to be there, it's your job, it doesn't cost you anything. You've got one tumour licked, but what about the metastases? Of course it's tempting to say, 'Let's have another go.' What have you got to lose? You'll be the hero. You're the guy battling ridiculous odds. You're the guy who has done eight operations on this person's child because you wanted to help. Aren't you *the guy*? But *are* you helping? And *who* are you helping?

I can understand how such selfless dedication to a lost cause could come across as a very self-affirming thing. A noble act. But actually, if the last six of those operations have been pointless, who are you doing them for? Are you performing them because you get kudos from it? I hope not. Is it so the parents can rest knowing they've exhausted all available avenues? Again, you probably shouldn't. Or perhaps it's because you haven't got enough gumption to tell the family that this is the end of the line? You've got a child who has maybe six months left on the clock. Have you wasted three of them in painful and ultimately futile procedures? Are you putting your own fear of delivering the truth over the well-being of your innocent but distressed patient? Do that and you're doing everyone a disservice.

It's a minefield. It shouldn't but it probably does depend on where a surgeon is in his or her own personal career. I've made my share of egotistical mistakes. But you only do each of them once. And the results are there forever. Today is not a day for ego.

'We're going to offer chemotherapy and radiotherapy to remove the last part of the tumour that we left in the head and also the spinal tumours. This will be starting as soon as he's regained his strength after the operation,' I explained. 'There is a small chance we can hold the metastases and treat them. But I can't see us operating on any of them.' It was Honesty 101.

'You say a small chance. How small?'

'The probability of your son surviving five years will be, even with maximum treatment, around ten per cent.'

Numbers can be harsher to hear than words. The woman was broken. When we'd first spoken, I was preparing her for the fact that her son was about to undergo serious invasive brain surgery. My mission then had been to make her aware of the risks concomitant with such a procedure. Patients can and do die on the operating table. I hadn't wanted there to be any surprises. But I hadn't prepared her for this. Just as I wasn't prepared for what she would say later.

· · ◆ · ·

I've been around a while.

Having these types of conversations is something that I've got a particular interest in doing, though not in a macabre way. I think that when you have people on whom you can't operate, it's actually where we as doctors, certainly as paediatric neurosurgeons, really come into our own. Of course, we can operate. But actually, it's about making people understand when operating is not the best option.

Imagine you're a parent. You have two choices: watch your child undergo a series of unpleasant physical chemical treatments that may or may not extend life or go home and enjoy the quality time you have left together. The relative chances of success of proposed treatments are presented to them, based on previous results, but we can't make any specific promises for their child.

Make no bones about it. Chemotherapy and radiotherapy are bastards. They're physically unpleasant. Hard labour for an adult, let alone an eleven-year-old. You can often come out feeling worse than when you went in. The logic is that it's short-term pain for long-term gain. Fine in a lot of cases, but what if you don't have a long term?

I'm never going to be the person who pushes science for the sake of it or enforce a treatment because 'it's what we do'. I will offer it and you can take it and I'll ensure it's delivered to the highest of standards. But I'll only insist upon it if there is a significant chance of long-term *or* high-quality survival. It doesn't need to be both, but one should be an aim at least.

What would be the benefit in this case? We are talking high-end tumour here. It's never going to release its grip on its victim. Between treatments the lad might be walking and talking, yes; but he'd be exhausted, constantly knackered, with side effects such as changing blood counts and multiple infections, while the inside of a hospital becomes his second home.

Would I push it for my own child? I can't possibly decide without being in that position. What I can say is that the potential benefits are pretty questionable. Is it a price you really want your child to pay? I often have these difficult conversations with an oncology colleague – a cancer doc – who is one of the people who have to treat patients with these poisonous drugs. They are the next crucial set of personnel after the operation is over.

And so what we say to parents is this: 'We've given you the facts. We've pointed out the pros and cons. Your child is probably going to die at some point because of this tumour. Ultimately it comes down to this: what sort of quality of life would you like for him/her in the time you all have left? It's your decision and we will support you either way.'

After the tears and the resentment and occasional outbursts of anger, the majority of parents concede defeat. Some of them choose treatment, some don't. And, as good as my word, we don't judge, we support. And then something like this comes along.

* * ✦ * *

It was the morning after the conversation from the night before.

'Thank you so much for everything you've done,' Mum said.

'Have you decided what you're going to do?' I asked.

It seemed that from her conversations with the nurses, she was opting for no treatment and quality of life, but I wanted to hear it from her, to make sure she understood the ramifications.

'Yes, I've decided.'

'You're taking him home?'

'No. I'm taking him to Germany.'

* * ✦ * *

You only have to flick through the ads in newspapers and magazines or type any ailment into a search engine and you'll find someone offering a miracle cure:

Losing your hair? Don't pay for expensive shampoos. Send us cash to learn the secret of keeping your thatch.

Got a loved one with Alzheimer's? Our book has the secrets you need for a full recovery.

Trouble in the bedroom? Send 50 bucks …

There's a fix for everything. We've all seen them. We've all probably ignored them or just laughed. So imagine how desperate you must be to not turn over the page one time, to not ignore their promoted adverts on your social media page. To look at those ludicrous words and say, 'You know what, I've tried everything else. What if they're right?'

So now we were in an interesting situation. I was offering Mum and her son six months of time with their whole family, in their own home, making happy memories – or a couple of years of hardship and crying and illness. Maybe (probably not), but maybe he would beat the odds, but endure all the side effects of the treatment. What I didn't seem to be offering was a lot of hope. Some parents need that more than anything else. And she'd found someone who was offering it in buckets.

He was in Germany. He was well established. He had a list of endorsements from previous patients on his website. He looked legit. *Except he promised to cure cancer with crystals.* Crystals.

To call it pseudoscience is being generous. Some practitioners believe that you can create a healing energy field around a patient using semi-precious stones such as opals, amethysts and quartz. Others place them on chakra points on the body and wait for the magic to happen.

Hogwash. Bunkum. Crap.

Using some types of alternative medicines, I can understand. 'Eastern' medicine, including acupuncture, has a rich history (in my ancestors' history, in fact) going back thousands of years, and has identified important pressure points in the body. It's an area of alternative therapy that still bears exploration. In other types of treatment, the positive psychological benefits can help some illnesses. But a needle or a firm knuckle into a pressure point to help joint pain is one thing. A shiny stone balanced on top of the skin to treat cancer? Give me a break.

Of course, that's not quite what I told Mum. 'How did you find him?' I asked.

'Google.'

'And you're sure he can help?'

'Honestly,' she replied, 'no, I'm not. But can you promise me that you can?'

She got me. Bang to rights. She knew I hadn't and I wouldn't promise her the outcome she wants. I couldn't. Based on science and medicine I could give her odds that she didn't like. I looked into her eyes and I knew she'd drop Germany in a heartbeat if I told her what she wanted to hear. My crime was not selling the product hard enough. I'm a doctor, a neurosurgeon, a father. I'm not a salesman. And I'm certainly not the snake-oil variety. But someone, it's clear, was selling something that this wrecked woman was desperate to buy. Which of course is the point. *She had to buy it.*

Perhaps I am being harsh on crystal therapy. Perhaps it does work. Perhaps it's only a matter of time before it's rolled out across the NHS. Perhaps, perhaps, perhaps. But you know what? Perhaps I'd have a different opinion if it were free.

'Do you mind if I ask how you'll be paying for this treatment?' I enquired.

She didn't pause. 'I'm going to put the house up for sale.'

Wow. It's worse than I imagined. 'But where are you going to live? You have three other children. What's going to happen to you all?'

She smiled. 'It's not about money.'

Oh no, I think, *that's where you're wrong. Money is exactly what it's about.*

I could have stepped in. I could have slapped down a long verbal pushback. I'm the expert. I'm Sir Lancelot Spratt. My word is law. To do that, though, I'd really, really need to believe I was offering the only viable solution.

There have been several high-profile cases recently which have gone beyond conversations between Mum and Dad and their eminent Health Care Giver, and have ended up being Parents vs Hospitals not only in High Courts but in every court above them. It was important to follow these cases to identify repercussions in my own speciality. However, as much as I could have punctured my patient's mother's dreams of foreign salvation – and I was seriously tempted to – it wasn't my place. At least so I thought.

It still haunts me. I didn't want to be the bad guy. I certainly didn't want to completely pull the rug from under this woman's feet. All I could do was emphasize again and again that her son was not going to survive because of these crystals, regardless of external promises. Her options as I presented them were to have the treatment we offered or let nature take its course – both choices were likely to end the same way. She would then bury her beloved son, the light of her life, and live a long, more sad but hopefully sometimes happy, life with her remaining children. Or, she could give all her worldly goods to some crook, *then* watch her son die and live an impoverished and self-flagellating life with three children who don't know why they're homeless.

Nothing I said made a difference. She realized that her actions were going to affect the rest of her life and the lives of her children. But for her it was worth it.

I wanted to say, 'Your son's as good as gone. Nothing can save him. But you can save his siblings. Surely it's what he would want.'

Any which way I explained, it sounded like I was completely stabbing Mum in the back. I couldn't help it. The longer it dragged on, the more blunt I became. Not because I want to win – there are no winners here – but because I cared for my patient *and* his family.

Their time at John Radcliffe ended a day after my patient was cleared for travel, ten days after his surgery. Which had given me ten days to test and probe Mum's mettle. To her credit, she never wavered. She wasn't aggressive or rude to us, she didn't apportion blame. If anything she was exceedingly grateful for everything we'd done or tried to do. But we were just one cog in the wheel. She was ready for the next turn.

· · ✦ · ·

It was about six months later that I received a letter from her. She thanked me, once again, for everything. She reported that the trip to Germany had been hopeful but ultimately unsuccessful. Her son had died peacefully at home three weeks earlier.

The brightest possible spin I can put on the whole episode is that the whole family ended their time together as a unit with an amazing overseas flight to Germany. It would have been an adventure. One final road trip for the entire gang. Something to remember everyone by. Forever.

Other than that, where were the positives? I knew the treatment wouldn't work. I knew we – or rather *they* – would still have a seriously ill eleven-year-old with a fatal condition at the end of it. But what really bugged me, what totally got under my skin was this: where was the family going to live when they returned from Germany? They'd sold their house. The charlatan with the crystals had taken everything from them; not just hope and common sense, but the roof over their heads. He'd sold a dream that couldn't be paid for, set a price that would affect so many other people's lives. I get it if you're a single parent with an only child. Maybe you'd risk everything. Walk over hot coals. Lay your own life on the line. But if you've got other children, other responsibilities, other dependants who need you for everything …

To this day I ask myself: should I have stepped in? Should I have insisted that Germany never happened? Should I have enforced textbook NHS care on that young chap?

My friends tell me not to beat myself up about it because it wasn't my fault. They say that the mum made her decision and I was powerless to stop her. But the truth is I wasn't. It was a choice not to interfere. Trust me, if I'd wanted to I could have caused problems for everyone. I'm a neurosurgeon, remember. I'm a disciple of James Robertson Justice. I have a God complex. And more importantly, I *do* have the power. Maybe I could have got an injunction, had her son made a ward of court, any number of things.

But it's not about me. It's never about me. The patient comes first. Win, lose or draw, that is the only statistic that matters. And sometimes nobody wins.

CHAPTER NINETEEN

IT'S NOT YOU, IT'S ME

W hat is success? I suppose it depends where you're sitting. The majority of my patients are like whirlwind romances. A relationship that burns bright but brief. They sweep into my orbit, I analyse, operate, repair and send them back out into the world. And that's it. In and out of my life, just like that. Perhaps I'll see them in clinic from time to time. Sometimes I won't. Their names, their memories, everything about them fades.

It's those other, special relationships, the ones that go on for a while, that you remember. They stay with you. That's not to say they are the ones where we've made a mistake or something has gone wrong. Some problems are just unfixable. You can slow down the effects of a condition, but eventually you're King Canute sitting on a throne in the sea, shouting at the tide to turn back. It doesn't mean you've failed. Even if that's how it feels.

It took me years to understand that success doesn't have to mean 'curing' or ensuring a patient lives forever. Sometimes success is just about making a difference.

· · ◆ · ·

Looking across my desk at the young girl in the wheelchair and her parents, it is hard to get too excited. She is frail, weak, exhausted and saddled with a horrible tumour. I'm not proud. I know I'm not her first 'date' – she's come to me via a surgeon at another hospital – but I am sure I am going to be her last. The question is: how long do we have?

She's got a craniopharyngioma, which is a particularly pernicious type of tumour that targets the middle of the brain. The fact that it's benign means nothing. It's located in a part of the brain that's very difficult to access and it is growing, albeit slowly. If it isn't removed she will die. Looking at her notes, looking at her, I'd guess within the year.

I explain everything to her. She seems chipper, she's accepted her lot. Her parents, unusually, are fairly chilled as well. You can see they all enjoy each other's company. If anything, coming to see me is a day out. It's great to see. So many mums and dads spend their last days with their children arguing or shouting or crying or locked away investigating various spurious Internet 'miracle cures'. It's understandable. It's human. But it's destructive. I'm sure they all look back and go, 'I wish I'd just taken the opportunity to enjoy being with my son for the little time we had left.' Come to think of it, that's good advice for me to take as well. And for you.

This family seems to have nailed it. They're taking each day as it comes and making the most of every second. I already love them. Which is why it's so disheartening for me to have to say, 'I honestly don't think we will ever be able to reach all of the craniopharyngioma. But if you'll let me, I'm willing to give it a damn good try.'

'That's all anyone can do,' Dad replies.

· · ◆ · ·

I operated multiple times. I spent days probing and burning and melting and vibrating and cutting. I wasn't doing anything her previous surgeon hadn't attempted, I'm sure. The difference was that month after month after month after month I was still trying. And I was prepared to keep at it for a long, long time, again and again. Whatever it took, as long as it was helping her.

Three years later, we were almost back to square one. Every time I grabbed a slice, a new piece grew back. It was like playing Whac-A-Mole, but rather more serious. She had radiation therapy which slowed the growth, but still it kept coming. We pretty much threw the kitchen sink at her and never made any headway. At best we were standing still, which actually was fine for my patient.

I watched her grow over those two, three, four, five years. She never got 'better' but she never got worse either. We were doing just enough to keep her stable, at a level she could manage. To watch her interact with her parents was a thing of wonder. They all carried on like nothing was wrong, like they weren't on the front line in an unwinnable war.

They enjoyed life and they revelled in it. Every day was an opportunity. A gift from God if they were religious; a new day if they weren't.

After every couple of operations we'd have the same chat: 'I'm going to keep on doing this for as long as you want me to. But there will come a time when perhaps the pain and discomfort and recovery time from surgery isn't worth it any more.'

'We know,' Mum replied. 'And we're grateful. But we're okay for now.'

And they were. We all were. Until that moment when we weren't.

· · ✦ · ·

It was our sixth year together. Things had been rocky for a while. The patient had stopped treading water, stopped standing still. Each operation, as far as I could discern, was taking more and more out of her. She was recovering, but much more slowly than before.

It's the same with some chemotherapy patients. The horrors of the treatment see a proportion of them quit the programme midway. They'd rather enjoy a few 'healthy' last months than endure a cycle of monthly torture/sickness/recovery/happiness/ torture/sickness/recovery/happiness.

This was the stage I felt we were reaching with my young patient.

'You know I'm willing to go again,' I said. 'You know I will always keep hunting. But I think the time has come to ask: is it worth putting her – all of you – through it?'

I didn't have to explain. Everyone in the room knew where we stood. For seven years we had kept a deadly tumour at bay due to regular invasive interventions. If we'd skipped any single one of those procedures, the craniopharyngioma would have taken hold completely and the girl would have been dead within five or six months. We kept fighting because she kept enjoying life. But now I wasn't so sure. Neither were her parents. And neither was she.

'One more try?' she asked, her voice feeble but clear.

'Of course,' I said. 'One more try.'

When we met six months later, everyone knew it was for the last time. And do you know what? We were all comfortable with that. I wasn't lying to the family when I said I'd fight their corner forever. I would. But after a while, once I'd realized that I was doing them no service perpetuating a young girl's suffering, I would have to recommend an end. And that was the point we were at. I knew it. The parents knew it. The girl knew it.

Honestly, though, even at that final clinic you would never have imagined what they had all been through. The mood was so light. Everyone so positive. I watched the little girl – not so little now – stare out the window as I was talking to her mum and dad.

'What are you looking at?' I asked.

'I'm just watching the way those birds are flying,' she said. 'They're funny.'

* · ◆ · *

Without further treatment, she finally succumbed to the tumour's unrelenting putsch six months later. I wasn't notified at the time, but a few weeks after that I noticed a familiar name in my clinic diary. When Mum and Dad came in alone, I knew what had happened.

I always encourage families to stay in contact with me after the passing of their child. As I've said, they are my patients as much as their son or daughter. My care – my interest – doesn't end with the completion of the surgical options. Mental wounds take longer to heal than physical ones.

'Thank you for letting me know,' I said. 'She was a wonderful girl. I'm sorry I couldn't do more.'

Mum was already in tears. Dad was close. 'We just wanted to pass on a message,' he said. 'She wanted you to know – she wanted us to tell you.'

I could see he was struggling. 'Tell me what?' I asked.

'To tell you that she was grateful for everything you did. Everything you tried.' He looked at his wife for support. 'And to apologize for making you feel bad that she never got better.' She may as well have said, 'It's not you, it's me.' It didn't stop me crying. Usually I wait until the patients or parents have left. This time I'm not sure I got away with it. To have that fortitude and even the inclination to think of others when you're literally at death's door was amazing. Her parents were just as impressive. There wasn't a hint of anger or regret or disappointment. Not directed at me, anyway.

'You gave us seven more wonderful years with our daughter,' Mum said. 'We will never be able to thank you enough.'

Nobody knows how they will react in adversity. 'Fight or flight' is a common phrase. But that's a very restrictive choice. The human mind is capable of so many other responses. As doctors you see a kaleidoscope of them, every shade, every nuance. Good or bad you have to deal with them all. And I think I have.

A different relationship was formed with an expectant family on another occasion. Mum had had a twenty-week standard ultrasound scan, and Baby was found to have a cyst on the brain. I spoke to both parents and gave them counselling about what could happen after the birth. The condition was serious enough for them to legally consider not proceeding with the pregnancy, but the decision had to be theirs. Based on my information they decided they wanted to go ahead. I could understand why. They were young – still in their teens. They were excited. They thought they had the world at their feet.

I attended the Special Care Baby Unit soon after delivery, as I try to do if I think there's a chance that emergency action might be necessary. From what I saw, we had a couple of days to play with. We could have been ready within a couple of hours if needed, but after months of stress and anxiety, Mum and Dad deserved some down time with their new one.

The cyst was in a very inaccessible location, smack in the middle of the brain. Tom Cruise in *Mission: Impossible* couldn't have airdropped in there without setting off the alarms. I kept the family informed of the risks.

'I won't know for sure until we get going, but from the scans alone I can't imagine I'll be able to get at more than a portion of the cyst.'

'What does that mean?' Dad asked.

'Probably that we will need to do this again before the year is out.'

It was just as I suspected. We put a lot of hours and effort into getting close to the cyst. Fortunately, Baby responded well to the treatment and we said goodbye – until the next time. The second procedure went just as well. Dad drifted off after about six months. They weren't married, and he found it too difficult to cope, I guess. That's the charitable view. The other view is this baby was getting in the way of his social life. I have seen it happen quite a few times with fathers. The maternal bond is undoubtedly the stronger one. Only once have I seen a mother disappear. That's another story.

Over the course of five years, I operated another seventeen times on this boy. I ended up having to put a shunt in to drain some of the cyst, and then open up other secondary cysts that appeared. For most of those times I was happy to continue. Each operation bought that baby and young mother a chunk of time to live and love and grow together without any problems. Eventually, though, the magic began to wear off. The law of diminishing returns had raised its head. The gap between procedures was getting shorter and shorter. After the nineteenth operation, barely six weeks since the last, I spoke to the mum.

'I'm not sure the treatment is working any more,' I said. She knew.

'I was worried you would say that. Aren't you going to help us any more?'

'Of course I will. You're both my patients. But we used to have four or five months in between surgery. Now it's down to five or six weeks. It's not going to get any better. You need to consider whether you really want your last moments together, your final memories, to be in this place surrounded by our machines, our people, our terrible décor.'

I didn't mention the fact that 'Baby' – as I still thought of him, even at the age of five – would be plumbed into those very machines. If I had a choice, I wouldn't want to see my loved ones leave this world like that.

Eventually, Mum reached a conclusion. When he was all set to go home after his final op, I said goodbye to my little guy, believing it to be the last time I would ever see him. And it was. Sort of.

Seven weeks later Mum called me. Her son had died peacefully in his bed in our local hospice, surrounded by his favourite toys and superhero posters. It was heartbreaking to hear.

'We'd be honoured if you'd come to the funeral.'

A funeral. For a boy I couldn't save. How could I go when I'd failed the whole family?

I can't think of many images in the world as distressing as the sight of a child-sized coffin. It goes against the very fabric of nature, of life and of hope. Being a stranger at a private function is awkward at the best of times. At a funeral, you feel like all the spare wheels in the world. The only people I knew were the family and they were there to bury one of them.

I was actually glad to be alone. If I'm honest, I felt like a fraud being there. I was the only one in the cemetery who had a chance of preventing the boy's death. And I couldn't. But that, it turned out, is not how everyone else saw it. Mum must have pointed me out to someone because a man came over, shook my hand and said, 'Thank you. Thank you for everything you did.'

He wasn't the only one. There was a procession of people, men and women, young and old, who wanted to show their gratitude for the time they'd got to spend with their little grandson or nephew or cousin or friend. 'Without you, we'd never have met him.'

But he died, I thought. *I couldn't save him.* Yet that's not what anyone there was thinking. To them it wasn't a life lost, it was five years saved. Where I saw professional failure, they only saw success, which made me smile on the way home. In between the tears.

And I made myself a promise. I will never attend a patient's funeral again. It's too tough, a price too high for me to pay.

CHAPTER TWENTY

THE CUSTOMER IS ALWAYS RIGHT

I'm in my office facing a husband, a wife and their eleven-year-old daughter. Two of them – the grown-up pair – are giving off the kind of warmth that even a snowman would find cold. Arms folded, lips pursed, eyes anywhere but looking at me. You'd think I'd killed their cat.

I'm used to a little more respect, to be honest. Admittedly, some people go overboard on the reverence. I'm not looking for that. I'd just appreciate people being prepared to listen to me. You know, considering they're the ones who've got the sick child.

I've seen their sort before, of course. Maybe not to this degree. But there are plenty who have crossed my doors who are either unreasonable in their expectations of the service I could provide or who just wanted things to happen immediately at their behest. The fact that I would have had at least another ten people to see, some of whom in more urgent need of treatment, mattered not one jot: 'Why can't you do the scan now? Why can't you operate now? I've got her pyjamas. Why would you delay it? You're playing roulette with our child's life.'

They're tricky to deal with. With most people I can say, 'I know you are anxious, I know you are worried, but I have dozens of other patients. Your child is safe – there is nothing that will happen suddenly and waiting will not make their condition worse. There are, unfortunately, some patients who cannot wait, and so are in your position but have been waiting for some time already. I have to prioritize. Try to look at it this way – it's always better *not* to be the patient that cannot wait because you are so sick … you want to be the patient that *can* wait.' That's usually the end of it.

But some people don't want to hear that. They shout, they rail, they threaten. You wonder what they do in their day-to-day lives. Are they bullies with everyone or just NHS staff? When your patient count is in four digits you get a sense of people, so I know what concerned parents look like. Shouting the odds doesn't prove a thing.

The truth is, scans aren't like Polaroids. Waiting lists for them can be approximately four-to-ten weeks, even longer for a scan under anaesthetic, which some people just cannot accept. I get that they love their child, but that doesn't make them experts in medicine and hospital procedure or more important than the parents in the next room or the room next door to that.

In this particular case, I sit across from them, waiting for one of them to break their pouty silence with something more than a curt 'yes' or 'no'. They had come to me for a second opinion from a very good colleague in another unit.

'Perhaps you can tell me why you decided to leave your previous hospital and come here?' I say. 'Your old doctor is probably one of the leading experts in this field.'

'He's a charlatan,' Mum replies. 'A fraud. A quack. A con man.'

Wow. 'Okay, why would you say that?'

'For a start, he said there's nothing wrong with our girl.'

'Interesting. And why do you disagree?'

'We googled it. She's got Chiari malformation. We demand treatment or we'll go somewhere else.'

Charming … Here is the rub. The notes from the previous hospital indicate there is a small Chiari malformation on the scan, but nothing serious. Certainly nothing that strongly correlates to the patient's symptoms. She's been sick and vomiting, but also angry and disturbed. There have been lots of behavioural issues. *And yet I can't take things for granted. I need to start with a clean slate …*

'Can I clarify that you were advised that Chiari is unlikely to be the cause of your daughter's problems?' I ask.

Mum folds her arms even more tightly and harrumphs. 'That's what the last idiot said, yes. He should be struck off.'

There follows five minutes of eviscerating abuse of a guy I know to be pretty solid at his job. Even if he weren't, he didn't deserve this abuse. No one would. 'Anyway …' I continue, 'did he tell you that surgery on your daughter is too great a risk for the possible benefits?'

'He was just making excuses.'

My turn to exhale. 'The brain is not something you operate on for the fun of it. Complications can occur, and these can be serious, rarely even life threatening. You really don't want to go there unless you have to.'

'Well, we think you *do* have to. And the customer is always right.'

'In a restaurant maybe, but in this room *I'm* the expert. You came here for my opinion about your daughter. You know her best, but I know what's best as far as the condition is concerned.'

'We don't think you do. We don't think you care about our little girl.'

Will it never end? 'Look,' I say, 'I'm not sure what you want to hear. My colleague from the other hospital seems to have conducted a very vigorous investigation. I've listened to everything you have said, and examined her top to toe. I'm inclined to agree with him. Your daughter might require an operation at some point in the future if things change, but certainly not now and possibly not ever. Her condition is extremely mild.'

'Oh yeah?' Dad responds, aggressively. 'So how do you explain the other problems?'

Oh, I wish you hadn't asked that. I have in front of me a ton of notes from psychology interviews conducted with the parents and the daughter. The key factor in all of it is that Mum and Dad are recently separated. Not that you could tell from the united front they're presenting against the old doctor and now against me, but I suppose the enemy of my enemy is my friend, etc.

The conditions they're complaining about started since news of the separation broke. What's more, the daughter's 'illness' seems to be quite virulent on weekends and holidays but absent when she's at school. It also appears to be quieter during time spent with Dad. Even I can see a pattern. Daughter blames Mum for the break-up, kicks off whenever she's in her orbit and relaxes a bit when she's not. Elementary, my dear Watson.

Except … Except there are physical complaints. Weakness, balance problems, headaches, swallowing difficulties, chewing issues, speech problems, double vision. She had reported all of them. Which is what, I suspect, has sent a series of doctors chasing golden geese.

Just for completeness, I order my own scans, which buys me a little time. In actual fact, I'm perfectly happy looking at a set taken by the previous hospital. They confirm mild abnormalities. Nothing, I would wager, that should result in the responses the daughter is reporting.

The last thing I want to do is throw this eleven-year-old girl in front of the bus. Especially a bus driven by her parents. But here's the thing: when children with functional problems are asked the same questions by different people at different times, they will often start to assimilate the inferences from the questions into their answers.

'Are you cold?'

'No.'

'Are you cold?'

'No.'
'Are you cold?'
'No.'
'Are you cold?'
'No.'
'How are you?'
'I'm cold.'

It's not necessarily misleading. It's just kids telling adults what they think they want to hear. I've seen a dozen patients who have parroted their symptoms straight from either the NHS online website or, more frighteningly, from Wikipedia. To be fair, Wikipedia sometimes has clearer definitions. Either way, it's a sad state of affairs when I have to check those particular sites before I meet a new patient in clinic.

The more I speak to the patient, the more contradictory her answers appear. I notice that she's taking prompts from Mum. Not only in the tricky stuff, but also quite straightforward questions like when I ask her when she first developed her symptoms. I see what's going on. I don't want to interfere. But I do want to help them.

Before I'm finished talking, the parents start chipping in with questions. A lot of them are irrelevant and nothing to do with me. Then, when they realize I've made my mind up, the questions become accusations: 'Why did we bother coming here? What a waste of time. You were supposed to help us. You're not a doctor, you're just a charlatan.'

It doesn't matter how many times I tell them their daughter is fine. Or that she doesn't need an operation. They won't listen. They don't want to. Dad launches into Mum, saying how the daughter should live permanently with him as she's clearly not happy with her. Then Mum tells Dad where to go, informing him how he's failed them both and how if he were a real man he'd sort me out.

Suddenly, Dad is up on his feet, towering over my desk. He's pointing at my face. Screaming at me. They both are. The door opens.

A colleague looks shocked to see this man mountain aggressively gesturing at me. He mouths the words, 'Should I call … ?'

'It's okay,' I say. 'I'm fine.' But for how long?

I stand up. Possibly the wrong move. I'm more than 6 foot. He's a good few inches taller. Wider. And he's furious. His face is so close I can feel his breath. Flecks of spittle bombard my skin. He's shouting the odds. Swearing. Telling me what he's going to do to me if I don't help his daughter.

I'm sure this tactic has worked on many people in the past. If I weren't quite so tall and not used to fairly aggressive behaviour in my social life, then I would feel quite worried. Maybe I'm too stupid to recognize the danger I'm facing. Or maybe it's because I survived Glasgow unscathed. You can be hit by anyone, of course. His wife is as likely to strike out as he is. Right now, he's my priority. I need to watch his fists carefully.

This isn't my first rodeo. Not my first threat of violence. I work in a very pressurized industry. I can normally talk them down. Bring them back from the brink of violence. I believe I can this time, but I don't get the chance to try. Mum suddenly decides she's had enough. She marches to the door and, dragging her daughter, demands that her ex follows suit. When they open the door, I see my colleague with two burly security guards. They step aside as the family storms past.

I never saw the family again. I pray they never found a surgeon willing to operate. Perhaps in years to come, that young lady will require surgery. But all she needed then was psychological help and parents who didn't want to kill each other, with her caught in the crossfire. Funnily enough, that wasn't mentioned in the letter of complaint they sent to the hospital …

CHAPTER TWENTY-ONE

YOU SAID THAT LAST TIME

No two days are the same. No two patients, nor their parents. Odd, really, considering how few brain complaints there actually are.

We were referred a baby – eighteen months old – from a hospital within our orbit. She'd experienced sudden onset collapse and seizure activity. Between me and my team we make a call on a) diagnosis and b) urgency. Judging from the scans that the hospital beamed over, we were looking at an arteriovenous malformation (AVM).

Collapses and seizures are a couple of the more time-sensitive symptoms for a lot of problems. We'd have to hit the ground running when she arrived. I was getting ready to leave for the night when the call originally came in. Three hours later, I was invested and ready to put in a night shift. Luckily, I wasn't alone. My registrar at the time – Tim (now a consultant himself) – was running around like a headless chicken getting the various departments prepped for our little visitor. I'd need scans, I'd need a theatre, I'd need nurses, equipment, anaesthetists, the works. Tim would handle procurement, of that I had no doubt. All I needed to do was call home and say I wouldn't be back for a while.

· · ◆ · ·

It's 10 p.m. Baby is twenty minutes away. I move our team up into the next gear. Without ward rounds and clinics and other distractions, we go straight to an abbreviated version of the WHO countdown.

'Okay,' I say, 'this is what we think we're dealing with, this is what I need – tell me how you can all help.'

Everyone else is as ready as me. Now it's just a case of waiting for the main attraction.

· · ◆ · ·

The parents arrive in a teary-eyed, tired bluster of panic. Ambulance trips can have that affect. I want to get the full history from them personally, but I let Tim lead the conversation. It's how registrars learn. It's exactly as the treating hospital explained. One minute the baby's fine, the next minute she's on the floor. Scans show a clot near the top of the brain.

I'm in the theatre running an eye once again over the scans. In the old days they'd all be pinned up on the walls, but in the computer age I get to look at them one at a time on screen then whizz forward to the next. It's cheaper than printing, I have no doubt, but far from as efficacious. Who has time to be flicking between images on a laptop?

We begin to prepare to do the blood clot/AVM treatment. When the anaesthetist wheels the patient in, I do another check of the room.

'Everyone good to go?' They are.

Fifteen minutes later, I'm inside her skull, cutting my way through to the blood clot. It's accessible. Not small – about 5 cm across. Fairly routine, I imagine, to take the majority of it out. My tools are arranged pristinely to my right. Tim's head is virtually touching mine as he keeps the entry points open. We are working as a seamless team, as would be expected after having him with us for six years. Behind him, our junior trainee's head spins between the screens, the heart monitors and ground zero. He's taking in everything. Exactly as I'd hope.

Occasionally, he'll have a question. I answer if I can. By that, I mean, I answer if the scenario allows me that luxury. If I'm working on a particularly perilous manoeuvre, that's where my conversation will stop. It's not personal. I probably don't even hear the question.

The priority is to remove the errant blood clot, while protecting the expected dangerous blood vessels underneath it. I've started on the operation, removing it piecemeal. Once I've got the area ready, I let Tim do some of the work, never taking my eyes off the clot.

We've been going an hour when he says, looking through the microscope, 'What do you make of this?'

I'm already looking at the giant images on the screen behind him. Something isn't right. The clot has been coming away beautifully. We've hoovered up nearly half. But Tim has hit upon something a little different.

'Shit,' I reply. 'I do believe we've got a Trojan horse on our hands.'

'I think so.'

It's what's peeping out from within the area that we're focused on. There's something else there. Clinging to the edge of the clot. I reach in with my instruments. I cut what I can and remove it with forceps. Tim studies it as I hold it to the light.

'Tumour?' he asks.

'Too right.' I show it to the rest of the room. 'I hope none of you had evening plans ...'

· · ✦ · ·

Talk about unlucky. This little girl had developed a tumour, which in turn had worn through a blood vessel, causing it to rupture. The tumour itself was barely different in appearance to the surrounding brain, so of course it's going to be overlooked on the scan, once the blood clot comes into play. The only positive from the situation was that the original hospital did a correct diagnosis. Just not a complete one.

The moment the tumour came into play, the whole emphasis of the operation switched. One minute you're prepared to do a vascular operation with certain instruments, suddenly you're on a different footing.

First things first: the scrub nurse packages a sample of the tumour. I say to the junior, 'Get this to pathology. Immediate turnaround. Any problems tell them to call me immediately.'

Off he runs. He has to get one of the pathologists in at this time of night, as they aren't paid to be on call any more. Cost efficiency and all that. But in these rare times, we rely on their good will to haul themselves out of bed and come in. They have never refused – true professionals.

In the meantime, we have two alien bodies to contend with. The clot is already looking like a pale imitation of the beast that had arrived. The tumour itself, once the surprise has been dealt with, isn't that intimidating. A brief pause, a quick pow-wow with the team and we are back in, only this time with different priorities.

What had been a straightforward clot removal became a tumour resection or 'debulking'. It goes smoothly. We get as much as we can. There are no hiccoughs. None that make themselves known during the operation, anyway. As always, the proof of the pudding would only become apparent when Baby wakes up.

It's a relief when she does. There's a weakness down one side – to be expected from our rooting around under the bonnet in what we call the 'motor strip' – the part of the brain that controls the opposite side of the body – but otherwise she's fine. If I had to put money on it, I'd guess she'll be back to normal within a couple of months.

Despite the hour, Baby's parents are wide awake when I find them. I don't think either had sat down for the last two hours, both still in shock about the blood clot. When I reveal the presence of a tumour, it's like I'd punched them in the stomach. Whatever adrenaline had been keeping them powered up disappears in a second.

'A tumour?' Mum says. 'Has she got cancer? Is she going to die?'

I explain that we've sent a piece off for analysis and also cut out as much as we could find. The problem was, because the brain was so angry from the clot, it had been hard to discern the edges of the tumour.

'We'll run some tests, we'll work out what we're dealing with and, if necessary, we'll go back in again when your daughter is strong enough,' I explain.

· · ◆ · ·

The news from the lab wasn't great. Baby had a glioblastoma, a very aggressive type of tumour. Even if you know it's there, it's a pretty hard one to treat. True to form, being a small child, Baby had enough about her to manage a solid recovery. Scans showed that we'd actually got rid of most of the tumour on the first sweep. Considering we hadn't even known it was there when we began the op, that was a pretty good result. But not perfect. And on this occasion, with this patient, I thought we had a shot at that.

Once all the swelling and angriness goes down, you can generally go back in and do a more controlled operation to really hunt out all the bits of the tumour that might be hiding away and resect – remove – as much as you can. We did that and took away as much as wanted to be found, and Baby underwent chemotherapy to take care of the more devious parts. It was three months later when I saw her again.

When the parents arrived for clinic they were shadows of the healthy young pair who'd originally walked in. I was desperate to give them some good news. Luckily, I was able to. Scans showed that whatever was left of the tumour was negligible.

'What does that mean?' Dad asked.

'It means you've got a period of quality family life ahead of you. Your daughter is a strong little girl. She's not giving up. Let's see how things go and get another scan.'

When they returned another three months later, there was a spring in their step. The scans had been good – no evidence of recurrence. Baby had continued to develop like any other toddler. It was great to see. She caused chaos wandering around my desk. Wouldn't sit still for a minute. I could tell Mum was getting agitated with her, but I wouldn't hear of it.

'Trust me,' I said, 'this is the best outcome I could wish for. Treasure the moments, please.'

They took me at my word. A further three months went by and again, clear scan results. Each time I saw them they were all buzzing with life, full of stories about where they'd been, what they'd done. My patient – this tiny thing that had been a step away from death when I first met her – was growing into a brilliantly cheeky little thing. It was wonderful to witness the progress. As a family, they weren't wasting a single minute.

Another three months passed and another. I began making plans to drop them back to a six-monthly schedule if the next meeting went as well. As much as I enjoyed their extremely upbeat visits, there was no point in letting them get worked up every quarter for no reason.

Unfortunately, we didn't get the chance to put the plans into action. It was not even a year after her initial presentation when we had to break it to her parents.

'I'm very sorry but the scans show the tumour is fighting back.'

'Is she going to die?' asked Mum. My little patient watched the conversation but was not involved in the decisions. She had grown up with these conversations all around her – the parents wanted it that way, but she didn't realize the gravity of the question.

'Not for a long time,' I said. 'Because we're all going to help fight this.'

Which of course we did. But going in for a second time was trickier than the first. Scarring on the brain tissue, from where I'd resected the tumour before, made identification nigh on impossible in places. Even with all of our devices – sat nav, ultrasound – it was really difficult to pick out tumour from brain.

In the end I had to return to basics, the old suck-it-and-see. I took small samples of the areas I was confused by and swiftly had them run up to the lab with the basic note, 'What do you think this is?' Then I'd poke around a bit more, working on the stuff I was confident about, before word came back. Sometimes the reply was 'We think this is a tumour'. Other times it was 'This looks like scar tissue and brain. Maybe just be a bit careful there.' There was a constant toing and froing between us and the laboratory, which of course adds to the pressure and really slows down progress. Thank goodness for the music keeping everyone focused. Good old Queen.

We got through it. It was, we all agreed, a good operation. Yet three months later, Baby was showing signs of weakness. The strong bounce back that she'd demonstrated after her initial operation wasn't there. Something was keeping her down. We repeated the scan. The tumour was reaching into new, deeper parts of the brain.

'It's by no means a foregone conclusion,' I explained to the family, 'I'm willing to have another look. I will try to get out as much as I can again.'

'Will it harm our baby?' Mum asked.

'It's a good question. I would never advocate surgery if it weren't necessary. The risks are high. But I don't think we have a choice here. Clearly the tumour's going to continue growing till it threatens her life otherwise.'

'If you're sure,' Dad said.

'I am. But I think we should all be aware that this will be the last time.'

The room fell silent. We all knew what I was saying. We were all aware that if I hadn't been able to get everything on the first and second pass, the chances of me getting lucky the following times were increasingly lower. But that wasn't the only goal. I also wanted to make space for the brain, as some of the effects of the chemotherapy she was having would cause the brain to swell. We did what we could knowing that it probably wouldn't be enough. Not in the long term. But that didn't mean we were out of options.

The next stage was some serious radiation treatment. My oncologist colleague suggested a new form of proton beam therapy which was showing very positive results when dealing with such a rapacious enemy. The only problem was that the technology was very expensive – and as a result there was none available in the UK.

It's one of the great things about the NHS that we, as practitioners, are encouraged to own our limitations. If we can't do something, we look around for someone who can. And so it is with treatment. If there's something that we can't provide because we don't have the equipment but which the NHS, with the expertise available, has decided would be beneficial, then we can pay for that treatment to take place elsewhere. The key point is that NHS experts – i.e. people like me – have to concur that said treatment will be beneficial. Basically, it's to stop us sending people to Germany for crystal therapy and the like.

And so it was that Baby and her parents jetted off to Florida. I think it went well. Certainly, as well as could be hoped. The tumour was kept in abeyance for a couple of years – and the family had a lovely time together.

Sadly, there's a reason we continue clinic appointments long after successful operations. Something as virulent as glioblastoma doesn't know when to quit. Nearly two years after the last sighting, scans showed a familiar scene. In truth, I suspected as much the moment I saw the family. That bright, bonny little bundle of energy wasn't herself. She was smiling and chatting, but I could see it was an effort. I couldn't gauge whether the parents were aware of the deterioration. When you're too close to something, you don't always notice the changes.

As only an occasional, albeit regular, viewer, I could tell something was off. She seemed listless when she wasn't hyper. Quick to drowsiness if she wasn't being spoken to directly. I wasn't, therefore, surprised when new scans showed the tumour was back and putting pressure on her brain.

We really wanted to avoid leaping back into the surgery route. There were some very interesting chemotherapy trials going on that weren't available when we first started our relationship some three or four years earlier.

'If you want I can speak to our oncology team running the studies and try to get you on-board?' said my oncology colleague.

The family never wavered. 'Show us where to sign,' Dad replied, positive as ever. 'Whatever this new regime is, if it buys us more time we'll do it.'

He hit the nail on the head there. As a parent he wanted nothing more than to share every possible moment with his young daughter. But he was clued up enough to know, after all this time, that length of survival wasn't as important as quality. As long as these new chemo trials weren't going to cause his daughter unnecessary or undue pain and discomfort, he and his wife wanted to try everything they could for their child. It's perfectly reasonable to me. Which is how I came to my next decision.

'In the meantime, while we're getting all the paperwork and logistics sorted,' I said, 'I'd like to have another look at this new growth. If I can take out as much as possible it will leave the chemo with less work to do. But this really will be the last time I go in.'

The whole family laughed. 'That's what you said last time,' Mum laughed. 'We'll see …'

She was right. I had said that and I'd meant it. I previously had seen no reason to subject her daughter to the repeated risk of surgery and the ordeal of recovery. What had changed? Well, my patient primarily. The difference between her normal bouncy self and the slightly deflated, listless version in front of me was distressing. I hoped if I could alleviate pressure on the brain then maybe she'd zip back to her usual self. On top of that, it made sense to have her as fit and strong as possible before embarking on chemo.

'One more try,' I said in conclusion. 'This is definitely the last time.'
'Yeah, yeah, yeah ...'

$$\cdot \quad \cdot \quad \blacklozenge \quad \cdot \quad \cdot$$

My whole focus during the operation is on making things better. Getting back that quality of life that I've witnessed over the last few years. I'm lucky to have known my patient during some wonderful times for her and her family. It shows me what potential there is if we get it right. It gives me something to aim for.

Unfortunately, the second we get inside I realize what we're up against. The new and improved tumour – tumour 2.0 – is stuck up against a large blood vessel in the middle of the brain. Debulking potential is going to be severely limited. The best I can do is to attack the centre mass of the malignancy. It's quite crude, using blunt force to remove the carcass of the tumour while leaving the edges to continue their perfidious journey into the brain.

None of it looks good. Not the tumour nor the probable outcome. The tumour is taking hold in the limbic system, the bit of the brain that deals with your personality and emotion. The part that makes you a person rather than a generic human and that makes this child her own unique self. There is nothing I can do to get to the parts already enmeshed inside her brain. I'm not going to risk overreaching. There's too much at stake. Even so, it will only be a matter of time before her memory and personality begins to alter and the little girl the family know and love starts to disappear.

Still, I'm not going to give up on her or her family. I get as much as I can out before calling it a day. 'Definitely the last time ...'

$$\cdot \quad \cdot \quad \blacklozenge \quad \cdot \quad \cdot$$

Except, of course, it wasn't. Six months into chemo, I saw another deterioration in the girl's personality, so I chatted with the family to ask if they wanted me to try once again to wrangle a few more good quality months.

They did. With the caveat, 'As long as you keep making her better, you keep going.' My thoughts exactly.

Unfortunately, while she did snap back into healthy mode as usual after the op, it was for a much shorter period of time. The tumour was just too embedded in the brain. To combat the effects of chemo, she was also on a ton of steroids so her weight had shot up. Combined with the personality changes at the next clinic visit, I barely recognized her physically or mentally.

When you get to the stage that a patient spends more time recovering from treatment than actually enjoying a decent standard of life, then it's time to ask who is really your priority? Because it's not the patient anymore.

I could see the way the wind was blowing. I spoke to my oncology colleague. The chemo hadn't been able to halt the onslaught in the brain, he said. The little girl was due for a second course imminently.

'Do you think she's up to it?' I asked.

The image of the lethargic, laggard, lifeless child waiting in my clinic filled our thoughts.

'Honestly,' he said, 'I'm not sure she is.'

We were both on the same page, although we'd taken different routes to reach it. I'm not sure how long I would have continued having 'one more try' with that little girl. When you saw how much difference each operation made, how buoyant and full of *joie de vivre* it made her for another six months or year, it was so tempting to keep plugging away. Like an addict: one more hit, one more hit. The harsh reality was that I was no longer buying a year's good health. It was a month, possibly a few weeks more if we were lucky. And even then, there were side effects. The radiant little tomboy I'd grown proud of probably wasn't, in all likelihood, ever coming back.

When I broke the news to the family, I told them that, in our opinion, it would actually be unethical to continue operating.

I wasn't sure how the parents would react, as they had been previously so gung-ho about pursuing every avenue, chasing down every medical possibility. Interestingly, though, they agreed with my assessment.

'We can see she's not getting better,' Dad said. 'We don't want to cause her any pain or discomfort for the sake of it.'

'We've had a good run,' Mum added. 'Now I think we need to accept it's coming to an end.'

It was exceptionally brave of them, incredibly mature. The way they adapted from being all-out pioneers to accepting the difficult situation and saying, 'Okay, our time's up' was impressive. But for them, as for me, it wasn't about the amount of time or the amount of life, it was all about the quality. They'd had seven wonderful years with a little girl who should, by rights, have never seen her second birthday. They knew that and they were grateful. As, I have to say, was the patient herself.

'If I don't need any more operations, will I see you again?' she said.

'Probably not,' I replied. 'Not unless I get an invite to your next birthday party.'

'Oh no, Doctor Jay, you're too old!'

The family returned to their local hospital, who were brilliant with supporting treatments. Then, when the time came, they took hospice care at home.

Of course it's sad that a little girl died. But, as the parents pointed out again and again, she should have gone nearly six years earlier. The blood clot in itself, if unchecked, would have been enough to do that. The fact that it took a second condition to kill her shows how strong – and lucky – she actually was. The way the little girl and her parents viewed it, every day was a bonus and they did their best to make the most of it.

So yes, although this child eventually died, we gave her five times the potential lifespan that was expected when she first arrived. We enabled her and her family to enjoy years of good memories, experiences and adventures together. Seven years might not be regarded as a particularly long life, but they made it all count and packed loads into their time together, squeezing out every last drop.

That's huge, isn't it? To be able to do that? To be able to play a part in it? To witness first-hand everything that makes us human at its very best?

I think so. I'm a very lucky man.

ACKNOWLEDGEMENTS

I love my job. I look forward to every day at work. I am in the rare position that there have only been two days in my consultant career where I have not wanted to go to work – those followed unexpected deaths of patients in the operating room, and so perhaps could be forgiven.

I have been privileged to have been let into the lives of so many extraordinary patients and their families, to help where I can. I am also afforded the chance to teach and train the next generation of doctors – all the time encouraging them to see the whole patient, not just the disease.

My thanks for this chance in life go to my parents and my big brother, who loved, protected me and moulded a rather wayward child. Also to my friends, medics and civilians, who keep me sane.

There is a whole team who look after my patients. It is obvious to anyone who has been in hospital that one doctor is pretty pointless without the rest of the group. Big kudos goes to my fellow paediatric neurosurgeons Shailendra, Amedeo and Tim, and my plastic surgery, oncology, anaesthetic, intensive care, paediatric and radiology colleagues who are the bedrock of the hospital that cares for so many of my patients. Eternal thanks to my nursing team on the wards and in theatre – where would we be without them? They literally keep my patients alive. There are play specialists who allay so many fears, psychologists, physios, occupational therapists and speech and language therapists who get my patients better after I have done my worst. And let's not forget all the porters, cleaners, cooks, housekeepers and managers who are all unsung heroes.

And, of course, lastly, my wife and three girls, who give me light in the darkest of times.

All of these people are everything that makes *me* human.